Skin Remodeling DIY

An Introduction to the Underground World of Do-It-Yourself Skin Care

By

Deborah Tosline

Skin Remodeling DIY

An Introduction to the Underground World of Do-It-Yourself Skin Care

by Deborah Tosline

Printed in the United States of America

First Printing, 2015

ISBN 978-0-9861807-0-5

Deborah Tosline Publishing

Phoenix, AZ 85020

This book is intended to be used as general information only and is in no way intended to replace medical advice, be used as a medical treatment program, diagnosis, or cure of any disease or medical condition. There are no warranties, expressed or implied, regarding the effectiveness of the practices described in this book. Products or substances discussed herein are for educational purposes only and are not intended as recommendations of the author or publisher.

To my daughter, Jacqueline, who believes in me, makes me laugh big, and loves me unconditionally; and to Scott whose brief presence graced me, thank you both. I am grateful for the many gifts of the world, without which I could not have written this book.

PREFACE

My education and work experience is in hard science, where hypotheses are tested through observation and experiments. I have two Bachelor of Science degrees: one in geology and one in ecology. I have worked in the fields of geology and hydrogeology for more than three decades. My approach to skin care is based on that scientific background and my love of research. My personal experience includes more than three decades of studying and practicing do-it-yourself skin care, a consistent facial exercise practice from 2002, and five years of teaching facial exercise.

When people ask me how I take care of my skin, they typically want to learn more about my methods. I wrote this book to explain basic concepts about the skin's structure and functions, and to introduce a variety of techniques that anyone can use to improve the quality of their skin.

CONTENTS

INTRODUCTION

Welcome to the underground world of do-it-yourself (DIY) skin care, a highly effective way to maintain and improve your facial skin and muscles. This book provides introductory information about skin care treatments you can use at home. I call it the underground or secret world of skin care because these methods are not readily available through mainstream media sources.

Cosmetic dermatology is a rapidly growing field that uses non-surgical methods to rejuvenate the skin. Generally offered by plastic surgeons, physicians at medical spas, and by estheticians at beauty salons, many of these same methods and treatments used by professionals can be adapted for home use to improve the condition of your skin and give it a refreshed and velvety appearance.

Current research shows that great skin is based on the premise of *use it or lose it*. Skin that is not stimulated regularly tends to thin, lose function and experience a decline in natural rejuvenation over time. This process can be slowed or reversed with the use of cosmetic dermatology treatments, which initiate a cascade of biochemical healing processes that promote the production of collagen and elastin. Integrating high quality anti-aging ingredients into your skin care products enhances this process. With time and repetition, the use of cosmetic dermatology treatments and skin care products that promote collagen production can result in stronger, thicker, and healthier skin that translates into the best looking skin possible!

As we age, face and neck muscles weaken, atrophy (shrink), and sag; the overlying skin also sags. Face and neck muscles can be strengthened and built-up with exercise. When facial muscles are exercised, muscle fibers break down and cause micro-injuries. Repeated over time, these micro-injuries heal and result in muscles that are stronger and more resilient.

Most of the current cosmetic dermatology treatments are supported by research. Other treatments that have not had clinical studies are typically supported anecdotally. When used consistently, these treatments can reverse skin aging and sun damage, stimulate new collagen production, soften or eliminate fine lines, eradicate age spots, and brighten dull skin.

Lifestyle plays a fundamental role in your health and, therefore, the appearance of your skin. Incorporating exercise, hydration, nutritious food, nutraceuticals, social interactions, stress reduction, and rest into your life and minimizing exposure to chemicals will result in benefits that include gorgeous skin.

This book is for you if you want to:

- save money
- minimize aesthetic dermatologist visits
- avoid surgical procedures
- supplement surgical procedures
- pursue a more natural skin care approach
- enjoy the convenience of at-home treatments
- manage your skin's aging process
- use premium active ingredients at a lower cost
- avoid synthetic chemicals and preservatives, or
- use high quality, DIY skin care products

This book provides introductory information on:

- skin anatomy and the skin's healing process
- ultraviolet sun rays
- how to make DIY skin care products
- examples of anti-aging ingredients
- how to enhance product penetration into the skin
- how to strengthen face and neck muscles and
- treatments to increase skin collagen and elasticity

After reading this book, you'll be able to use simple DIY skin care techniques to improve your skin and facial muscles and you'll also have the information you need to pursue more complex facial treatments.

....

Tip: Use a microfiber washcloth when cleaning your face to remove dead skin cells and stimulate your skin; make a simple revitalizing vitamin C serum and use it daily to brighten skin; practice three quick facial exercises daily and a five-minute facial lymphatic massage weekly to strengthen muscles and reduce puffiness. Start this introductory level routine and move on to advanced ingredients and skin care tools to minimize the effects of damaged skin and achieve amazing results.

BACKGROUND

Some of the DIY skin remodeling techniques described in this book, and the associated gadgets and tools, are not well known. For example, the dermarolling technique—professionally referred to as percutaneous collagen induction therapy (PCIT)—was developed in 1996 by South African plastic surgeon Desmond Fernandes. In 2007, when I began dermarolling, the technique was not typically offered by dermatologists or at esthetician clinics.

In fact, I met a plastic surgeon in 2011 who told me that he was the only dermatologist in Tucson, Arizona, offering dermarolling at that time. Thus, it is not uncommon to encounter estheticians, dermatologists, or even plastic surgeons who may not know much about the treatments described in this book and may not be able to advise you about the use of them. However, the research is available if one knows where to search. The Internet is also a great way to learn more about the underground world of DIY skin care and locate folks who share their experiences about using DIY skin care treatments at home.

Tip: Check skin care Internet boards such as http://www.essentialdayspa.com/ forum/ for discussions about new and existing do-it-yourself skin care techniques, ingredient and device reviews, new recipes, and more. The information on these boards is available months or even years before it is published in mainstream media.

COSMETIC DERMATOLOGY

The overall result of cosmetic dermatology treatments is smooth skin that has a glowing appearance.

Cosmetic dermatology uses a combination of treatments to improve the condition of aging skin including, but not limited to: micro-current, light-emitting diodes (LED), lasers, dermabrasion, dermarolling, and radiofrequency devices. All of these processes work by wounding the skin, which triggers a biologic healing cascade associated with skin remodeling processes to produce collagen.

To impact different layers of the skin, cosmetic dermatology treatments or devices may be used at varying intensities. Low-intensity treatments primarily target the shallow layers of the skin and require little to no recovery time. Higher intensity treatments target deeper skin layers and require longer recovery times but result in more collagen production.

Cosmetic dermatology treatments also contract and tighten skin tissue. The contraction provides the foundation for new collagen production over a period of up to six months following the treatment, which, studies show, results in new and visible collagen production. The formation of new collagen fibers results in thicker skin. It should be noted that improvements vary by individual and may be somewhat unpredictable with sun-damaged skin.

Minor side effects may be experienced after cosmetic dermatology treatments such as red and inflamed skin. This condition is usually minimal, disappears after a few hours or, for some treatments, a few days, and can be hidden with a good makeup concealer. Extensive skin damage can be treated effectively using aggressive cosmetic dermatology treatments; however, aggressive treatments require longer recovery times.

Incorporating a single new skin care treatment into your routine is beneficial and, with time, your skin condition will most likely improve. When you integrate several different skin care treatments into your routine, the combination produces a synergistic, or combined, effect that is more noticeable than individual treatments done separately over time.

Tip: Use a microdermabrasion device periodically to exfoliate dead skin cells and encourage new skin cells to form, to brighten skin tone, and refine pores.

Adding another treatment, such as ultrasound once a week, further enhances new collagen development.

COSMECEUTICALS

The term cosmeceutical generally refers to a product created by combining a cosmetic with a pharmaceutical, or drug that is designed to promote biologic activities that improve the skin.

Cosmeceuticals consist of vitamins or other active ingredients such as antioxidants, minerals, proteins, enzymes, hormones, acids, and herbs that are added to skin care products. Some cosmeceuticals require prescriptions, such as certain forms of vitamin A including retinoic acid or tretinoin.

Studies have shown that retinoids, hydroxyacids, and some antioxidants have a positive impact on collagen production. While the effectiveness of many anti-aging ingredients, or actives, is documented by users' anecdotal evidence, clinical studies have not been conducted on all actives to support these claims.

DIY cosmeceutical skin care products may be used alone to nourish the skin or in conjunction with cosmetic dermatology treatments to enhance skin rejuvenation and promote skin remodeling. For example, vitamin A, vitamin C, and peptides like palmitoyl pentapeptide-3 or matrixyl play a vital role in promoting healing and in optimizing collagen and elastin production when using skin rejuvenation tools. Alpha lipoic acid has been shown to enhance the effects of cosmetic dermatology laser treatments.

Tip: Make an easy recipe for glucosamine/niacinamide serum and use it every morning after you wash your face. Let it soak in—or not, depending on your schedule—before applying other products. This serum will minimize brown spots and nourish the skin. You can easily buy the ingredients from an Internet store.

SKIN BIOLOGY

The skin is an organ comprised of three layers: the epidermis, the dermis, and the hypodermis or subcutaneous fat layer.

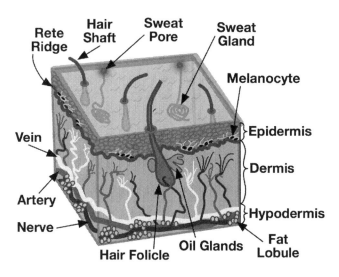

Layers of the skin

EPIDERMIS

The epidermis is the outermost layer of skin. The thickness of the epidermis depends on where it is located on the body. It is thinnest on the eyelids and thickest on the palms and soles of the feet. On the face, it is about 0.1 millimeters, about the width of a human hair.

The epidermal layer is comprised mostly of keratinocytes, which produce the fibrous protein keratin that protects the epidermis. There are three specialized cell types found in the epidermis:

- melanocytes, produce the brown pigment melanin
- Langerhans cells, involved in immune response
- Merkel cells, involved in nerve responses but their exact function is unclear

The epidermis itself contains five levels:

1. stratum corneum (top), made of dead skin cells that shed
2. stratum licidum, found in the fingertips, palms, and soles of the feet
3. stratum granulosum, site of keratin formation
4. stratum spinosum, provides strength and flexibility to the skin
5. stratum basale (bottom), forms new cells, basal cells

The epidermis protects your body and internal organs and is the first line of defense against infection.

The stratum corneum consists of horny skin cells held together with lipids (fats), similar to the construction of a brick wall. The horny skin cells act as the bricks and the lipids are like the mortar that holds them together, resulting in the formation of a protective barrier.

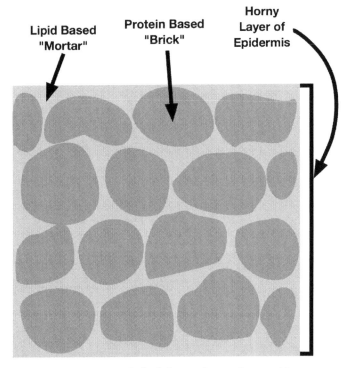

Lipid Based "Mortar" **Protein Based "Brick"** **Horny Layer of Epidermis**

Stratum corneum's brick and mortar pattern

All the cells in the epidermis originate from the base of the epidermis layer. As new cells are formed in the base they push previously produced cells upward. As the cells make their way up to the top layer, they become flattened and die. The production of new cells is a continuous process.

Dead skin cells are shed from the epidermis daily—a process that slows as we age. Exfoliating dead skin cells promotes the production of new skin cells. It takes three to five weeks for a skin cell to move from the bottom of the epidermis to the stratum corneum and skin surface. The health of the skin cells in the epidermis is dependent on the nourishment received from the layer below, the dermis.

DERMIS

Beneath the epidermis is the dermis, or dermal layer, of skin. The primary cells in the dermis are fibroblasts. The primary function of the dermis is to sustain and support the epidermis. To that end, the dermis, which is 10 to 40 times thicker than the epidermis, contains several specialized structures such as:

- hair follicles, formed by the epidermis and dermis
- sebaceous glands produce the oily substance sebum
- scent glands
- eccrine and apocrine sweat glands
- blood vessels carry oxygen, nutrients and wastes
- nerves transmit sensations such as pain and temperature

The dermis is made up of three types of tissue that are evenly distributed:

Collagen is a type of fibrous protein that connects and supports other body tissues. It is one of the most common proteins in mammals; more than 25 types of collagens occur naturally in humans. Collagen is sometimes referred to as the glue that holds the body together.

Elastic tissue is a type of connective tissue that gives skin the ability to stretch and then return to its original shape.

Recticular fibers are a special connective tissue, also known as collagen type III.

The dermis has two layers. The upper, closest to the epithelial layer, is called the papillary, which contains a thin coat of collagen fibers. The lower layer is the reticular, comprised of a thick arrangement of collagen fibers positioned perpendicular to the skin's surface.

The dermis contains many specialized cells and structures. The sebaceous glands produce natural oils called sebum. It travels to the surface of the epidermis to keep skin lubricated and protected. It is the substance that makes skin waterproof. When sweat, which is produced continually, emerges from the pores in your skin, it combines with sebum to form a protective film.

DERMAL-EPIDERMAL JUNCTION

The junction between the epidermis and dermis is an important structure that interlocks the two skin layers together with fingerlike projections called the rete ridge. Folds in the rete ridge increase its surface area, ensuring that the epidermis receives the maximum amount of nutrients from blood vessels in the dermis.

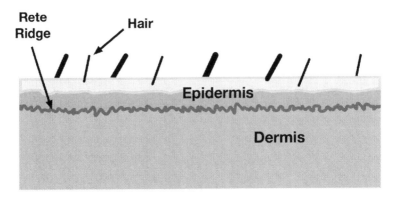

Rete ridge between the epidermis and dermis

HYPODERMIS

The hypodermis is located beneath the dermis and consists mainly of subcutaneous fat that protects deeper tissues. This layer contains collagen, elastin, nerves, and blood vessels that supply oxygen and nutrients to the skin, as well as lymph channels that carry wastes away from the bloodstream.

PH

pH is a measure of acidity and alkalinity based on a scale of 1 to 14 from most acidic to most alkaline. Human skin is fairly acidic, which helps it ward off harmful bacteria and fungi. Bacterial enzymes continuously break down the fatty acids to maintain the pH of the skin between 4 and 6.75 and buffers alkaline products that have a pH between 8.0 and 10.5. The optimal pH for human skin is 5.5.

Human skin has an outer, protective layer called the acid mantle, a thin acidic film that keeps bacteria out of the skin cells. The acid mantel is comprised of a layer of fatty acids that form an oily substance secreted by glands that keeps the skin from drying out.

Skin care product recipes rarely list pH testing as a routine step. One exception is homemade vitamin C serum, which recommends testing to ensure its pH is between 2.5 and 3.3. This pH level enhances absorption of vitamin C into the skin. Acid peel products, such as salicylic or glycolic acid, are applied to the skin in cosmetic dermatology and may be described by their pH levels.

A simple way to measure the pH of a product is to use a paper pH strip purchased from a drug store.

....

Tip: Use microdermabrasion or glycolic acid peels to treat the epidermis and ultrasound or a deep dermaroll to treat the dermis. Combining treatments can result in noticeable improvement in the condition of the skin including collagen and elastin rebuilding for thicker, more resilient and glowing skin, refined pores, and even skin tone.

LYMPH SYSTEM

The lymphatic system is present throughout the body. It transports and filters wastes from the bloodstream for processing by the liver. The lymph system does not have its own pump system; instead, it relies on physical activity to promote circulation. If you are inactive, the lymphatic system may not function properly and wastes may accumulate, resulting in puffiness in the face and neck. For example, under-eye bags may be due to poor lymph circulation.

There are a variety of ways to promote lymph circulation: physical exercise, facial massage, skin rejuvenation treatments, and dry brushing. When I began using facial lymphatic massage as a part of my routine, my under-eye bags disappeared.

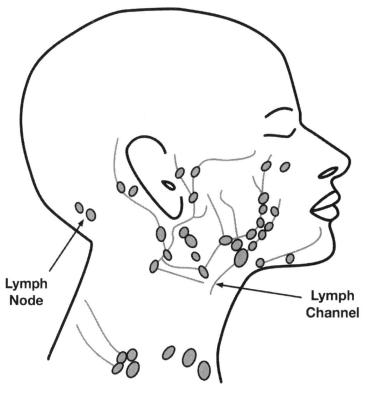

Lymph Node

Lymph Channel

Lymph system of the face

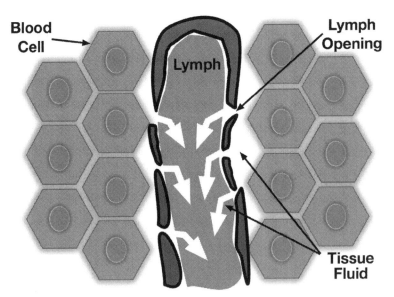

Movement of waste into the lymph

Tip: Use a facial lymph massage to eliminate under eye puffiness. Begin by massaging daily for two weeks and then once a week for maintenance. It takes five minutes and it is effective.

FACIAL MUSCLES

There are dozens of muscles in the face and neck. The muscles of the face control movement of the skin and other muscles when making facial expressions.

Facial muscles are structurally different from the muscles of the body. Below the neck, both ends of a muscle are attached to bone. Facial muscles attach to the bones of the skull on one end and attach to other muscles or skin at the other end.

Exercising facial muscles helps to retain or increase muscle strength, supports the overlying skin, increases skin circulation by 10 times, and stimulates collagen production.

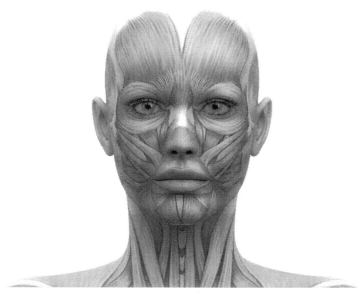

Facial muscles

© Decade3d, Dreamstime.com, Female Head Muscles Anatomy - Front

Tip: Practice resistance facial exercises to keep your cheeks and lips full, your forehead lifted, and your chin strong all while minimizing skin sag. The increased circulation will make your skin glow. Do this forever!

SKIN AGING

Typical signs of skin aging include: development of deep dynamic wrinkles that appear when facial expressions are made, loss of facial fullness, loss of tone, sagging, and photo-damage. As skin ages there is a reduction of nerve endings and blood vessels and the production of nutrients is reduced. As a result, the epidermis and dermis become thinner and lose elasticity. As the skin thins, it becomes more susceptible to damage and heals slower. Collagen helps maintain skin thickness; however collagen production decreases with age, resulting in thinner skin.

Skin aging is a result of intrinsic and extrinsic factors. Intrinsic factors are associated with genetics; extrinsic factors include sun damage, smoking, and exposure to chemicals. Extrinsic aging is believed to cause 90 percent of all skin aging.

With time, habitual facial expressions break down muscle fibers resulting in wrinkles that remain after an expression is made (static wrinkles) as opposed to wrinkles that disappear after a facial expression is made (dynamic wrinkles). Even the nose is susceptible to aging: ligaments and skin elasticity in the nose weaken with time so the nose becomes longer.

When facial muscles weaken and sag, the overlying skin sags as well. For example, as the cheek muscles atrophy or become less full, folds form in the overlying skin. The lines that form from the nose to the mouth are referred to as nasolabial lines. These skin folds are preventable if facial exercise is used to keep the muscles beneath the skin strong and full.

Skin aging is also the result of free radical damage. Free radicals are unstable and reactive molecules that may result from trauma, infection, inflammation, oxidative stress from byproducts of normal cellular function, and from environmental conditions such as pollutants. Free radicals generate collagenases, enzymes that degrade collagen and damage skin on a cellular level as they accumulate. This results in degradation of the skin, causing it to lose its youthful appearance.

Physical changes in the aging epidermis include flattening of the rete ridge between the epidermis and the dermis and a loss of fats in the hypodermis. When the rete ridge flattens, the result is reduced nourishment to the epidermis. A flattened rete ridge also causes the skin to become more fragile.

Aging occurs in each layer of the skin including the epidermis, dermis, and the hypodermis tissues. A holistic or comprehensive skin care program uses a variety of treatments to address aging in each of the skin's layers.

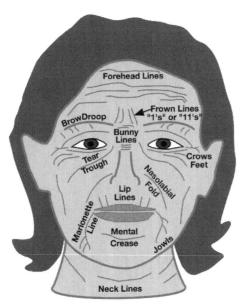

Deep lines that commonly form during aging

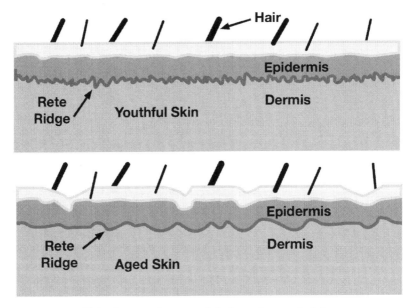

Skin layers in youthful and aged skin

Tip: The least expensive, most effective option to maintain youthful skin is to protect it from the sun. Small exposures over a lifetime matter so make a habit of covering your face, neck, and chest with a pretty scarf when you walk through a parking lot to maintain unblemished skin. Wear gloves to protect your hands when you drive. Use a vitamin C serum daily to protect and revitalize the skin.

HYPERPIGMENTATION

Skin discolorations that are brown, red, or yellow are referred to as hyperpigmentation, melasma, sunspots, or freckles and result from the over-production of melanin by melanocytes. These are specialized cells located at the base of the epidermis.

When the skin is exposed to UV light, melanin migrates and concentrates to absorb those wavelengths and protect the skin from damage. Hyperpigmentation may result from pregnancy, oral contraceptives, hypersensitivity, and sun exposure. One line of defense against hyperpigmentation is to reduce exposure to ultraviolet rays. Certain skin care ingredients suppress melanin production to reduce the production of dark pigments that cause hyperpigmentation.

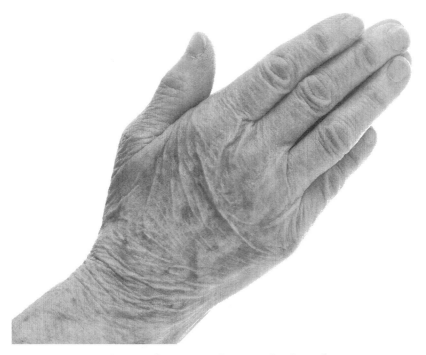

Hyperpigmentation on the hand

Tip: To prevent, reduce, or eliminate hyperpigmentation use a glucosamine/ niacinimide serum and afterwards, a vitamin C serum daily; wear sunscreen rain or shine, every day; and use clothing and shade to protect your skin during sun exposure. Take it a step further and use cosmetic dermatology devices to further enhance the beautiful results.

SKIN REMODELING

To keep skin looking healthy and youthful, it is important to promote cell turnover by exfoliating (removing) dead skin cells from the epidermis to ensure optimum penetration of cosmeceuticals and by using skin remodeling techniques to enhance collagen and elastin production in the dermis. Current skin remodeling techniques are based on the concept of inflicting micro-injuries to the skin to increase collagen production, which makes the skin stronger.

The micro-injury concept is similar to muscle building. Exercise works the muscles to fatigue, which results in small tears or micro-injuries. When the micro-injuries heal, the muscle is stronger. When a micro-injury is inflicted in the skin, a cascade of biochemical reactions immediately occurs to repair the wound. Studies focusing on wound healing have shown that growth factors accumulate at the wound site and work together to promote healing, including the production of collagen, resulting in thicker skin.

Wound healing involves three phases:

1. *Inflammatory:*
   begins immediately following the micro-injury
2. *Proliferative:*
   a rapid increase in tissue formation that begins about five days after inflammation and lasts about eight weeks
3. *Remodeling:*
   biochemical healing processes lasting from eight weeks to one year

Twenty-eight types of collagen have been identified, including:

- **collagen I**: skin, tendon, vascular ligature, organs, bone
- **collagen II**: cartilage - main component
- **collagen III**: reticulate fibers - main component, commonly found with Type I
- **collagen IV**: epithelium secreted basement membrane
- **collagen V**: cell surfaces, hair and placenta

Approximately 90 percent of collagen in the human body is Type I. Types I and III are often discussed in facial skin remodeling.

In the early phase of healing, Type III collagen is produced and reaches its maximum production in about five to seven days. Longer initial inflammation phases result in increased Type III collagen production. Following an injury, tissue remodeling continues for months as Type III collagen is replaced by the stronger Type I collagen.

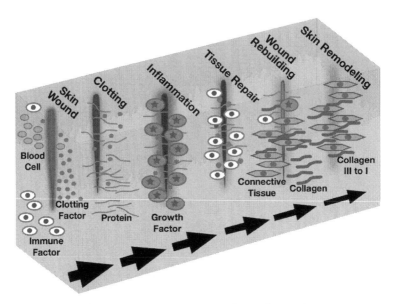

Biochemical processes after skin injury

. . . .

Tip: Use methods to promote the healing process and to promote collagen and elastin production after do-it-yourself cosmetic dermatology treatments. Use Retin A or retinol every night and a vitamin C serum every morning. If you have completed an advanced facial, use an oil soluble serum with a combination of retinol and vitamin C. This non-irritating serum provides ingredients necessary for skin rebuilding.

SUN EFFECTS

The rising sun makes for a wonderful start to each day. Its warmth on the skin is undeniably appealing. However, if you want your skin to remain youthful, you must develop habits to always protect your skin from ultraviolet (UV) sun exposure. Research has shown that 80 to 90 percent of UV radiation occurs during short-term exposure, such as when you walk from your car through a parking lot or driving to and from work.

It is easy to see that the most effective beauty routine is to protect the skin from sun exposure; Look at the skin on your body that is rarely exposed to the sun. It is probably unblemished and smooth.

Sun exposure accounts for an estimated 90 percent of premature skin aging or photo-damage. This damage occurs because the sun generates free radicals that break down the collagen and elastin structure in the skin resulting in sagging skin, an irregular skin surface, wrinkles, a thin and flattened rete ridge, irregular brown pigmentation, and skin growths.

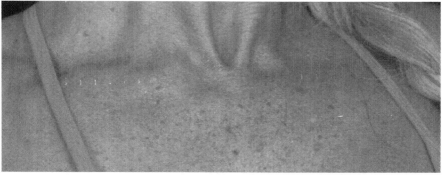

Sun damage on the chest

As mentioned previously, sun damage to the skin is an example of extrinsic aging. Extrinsic skin aging results in densely packed collagen that lacks elasticity. In photo-damaged skin, the elastic connective tissue beneath the epidermis and dermis is degraded and results in uneven skin texture and wrinkles.

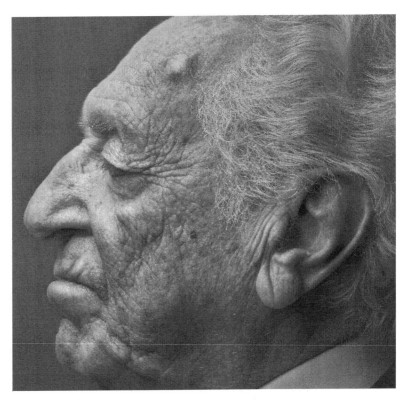

Sun damage

UV exposure increases enzymes that degrade collagen. For comparison purposes, it has been reported that the thickness of the dermis decreases up to 20 percent in skin damaged by the sun; however, in sun-protected skin not only is this same 20 percent decrease in collagen delayed until the age of 80, but there is also only a minor degradation of elasticity up until the age of 70 years.

SOLAR RADIATION

The radiation in sunlight includes UVA and UVB wavelengths as well as infrared radiation (IR), which is not visible but can be felt as heat waves.

UVA and UVB are both harmful, so use a sunscreen that protects against both. To make sure you're getting effective UVA as well as UVB coverage, look for a sunscreen with an SPF of 15 or higher, plus some combination of the following UVA-screening ingredients: stabilized avobenzone, ecamsule (Mexoryl), oxybenzone, titanium dioxide, and zinc oxide. You may see the phrases **_multi spectrum, broad spectrum,_ or _UVA/UVB protection_** on sunscreen labels, and these all indicate that some UVA protection is provided.

Apply sunscreen daily, rain or shine, to your face, neck, chest, hands, and any other exposed skin.

UVB rays penetrate the epidermis, causing sunburn and, with time, photo-aging. UVB rays are at their strongest during the middle part of the day.

UVA exposure penetrates the dermis and results in deep skin damage and photo-aging. UVA rays have the same damaging strength from dawn to dusk.

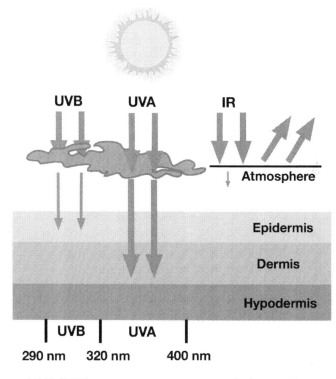

UVA/UVB spectrum, range and absorption

Cloud cover blocks most UVB rays, but 90 percent of UVA rays pass through clouds. UVB and UVA rays suppress the immune system, which reduces the body's ability to protect itself from cancer.

When IR light is combined with UVB and UVA exposure, it also encourages photo-aging.

SUN PROTECTION

Extrinsic photo damage is one of the largest contributors to skin aging. The most effective treatments for protecting your skin from sun exposure are daily use of sunscreen and specialized photo-protective clothing that covers your face, neck, hands, and chest from the sun. Sun protective clothing is now commonly available at outdoor sports stores, retail stores, and on the Internet.

Even everyday clothes such as tightly woven hats, long clothing, and gloves protect your skin from sun exposure. You can also lower your sun exposure by using a parasol or umbrella to shade your skin when you walk in the sun.

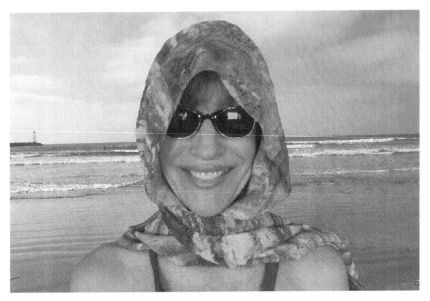

Use a scarf for sun protection

Currently, there is a debate over the use, effectiveness, and hazards of sunblock versus sunscreen.

Sunblock uses titanium and zinc oxides to physically scatter UVA, UVB, and IR rays. These products may leave a whitish cast on the skin but are desirable because they contain fewer ingredients and chemicals. Some products contain oxides that are broken down into smaller particles making them invisible when applied to the skin. In general, for people with skin allergies, it is best to use a physical sunblock to minimize allergic reactions.

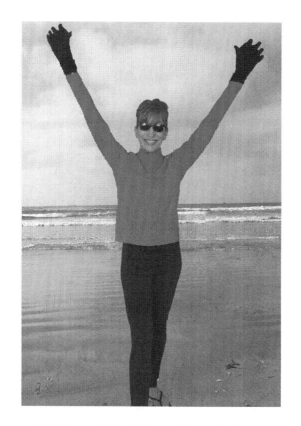

Full length bathing suit and gloves

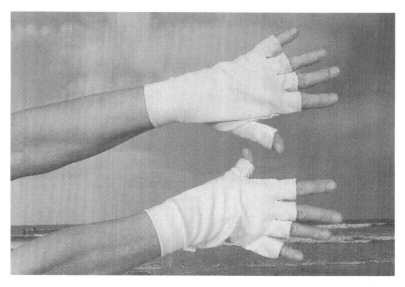

Sun protection gloves

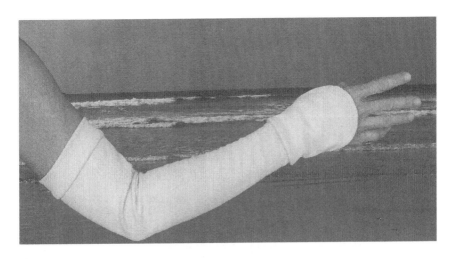

Sun protection sleeve

Sunscreens blend into the skin when applied and consist of synthetic chemicals that absorb UV rays. A chemical sunscreen with an SPF of 20 or greater typically contains chemical UV absorbers that can cause allergic reactions.

Currently available UVB sunscreens absorb the full UVB spectrum, but UVA sunscreens primarily absorb only the shorter UVA wavelengths and therefore, may not provide complete UVA protection. The most complete UVA coverage is obtained with sunblocks that contain a combination of titanium dioxide, micronized zinc oxide, and the synthetic ingredient avobenzone. Be sure to reapply regularly; studies show that avobenzone can degrade within one hour of sun exposure and lose its ability to block UVA wavelengths.

Although avobenzone is generally well tolerated, it can cause allergic reactions in some people.

Antioxidants like vitamin C, vitamin E, and ferulic acid also provide protection against sun damage. A 15 percent solution of vitamin C blended with 1 percent vitamin E and 0.5 percent ferulic acid results in a four- to eight-fold increase in sun protection. Apply these antioxidants during your morning skin care routine before applying sunscreen, or purchase sunscreens that contain antioxidants for added protection against photo damage.

Tip: Carry an umbrella and use it rain or shine, dawn to dusk. Use an umbrella when walking across parking lots, to nearby cafes, or when doing errands. When appropriate, an umbrella may be used to protect your skin from the sun while avoiding "hat hair." Remember that short exposures count, so make a habit of covering up as often as you can.

LIFESTYLE

While cosmetic dermatology and cosmeceuticals can significantly improve the condition and appearance of your skin, the best foundation for beautiful skin is good nutrition and a healthy lifestyle.

Detailed information about nutrition and exercise is readily available on the Internet, in magazines, and from the library. Everyone should take the time to learn more ways to enhance healthy lifestyle practices. That said, this section includes a summary of my personal observations and opinions of what a healthy lifestyle is, and general recommendations on how to achieve it.

When you make a choice to eat high quality food, hydrate with water, exercise regularly, minimize your exposure to chemicals, maintain a positive attitude, develop a good social network, get sufficient relaxation, and good sleep, you approach skin care from a holistic or broad perspective. If you are not currently living a healthy lifestyle, start slowly and make small changes that are easy to integrate into your routine and feel comfortable to you. Developing and maintaining a healthy lifestyle is an on-going process that can benefit you, your family, friends, and the earth!

NUTRITION

Thanks to mass media and digital communication, Americans appear to be more aware about healthy eating than ever. But the mainstream diet in the United States has become inherently unhealthy: look at the increased incidences of obesity and Type 2 diabetes in adults and children. These conditions are preventable through diet and physical activity.

Once you know how to make truly healthy food choices, eating becomes more than basic nutrition; it transforms into a gourmet feast of delicious, rich, and wonderfully nutritious super foods.

Organic and Local Food

Organic foods, i.e., food grown and produced without chemical and synthetic pesticides and fertilizers, irradiation, sewage sludge, antibiotics, synthetic hormones, or genetically modified organisms (GMOs), have been a staple of my diet since 1990.

Choosing to buy organic allows me to minimize ingestion of chemicals by my daughter and myself and to protect the environment by supporting sustainable agricultural technologies. Try to buy local whenever possible. Buying locally supports the local economy, reduces the travel time of perishables, and reduces the energy required to transport food.

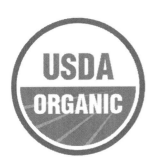 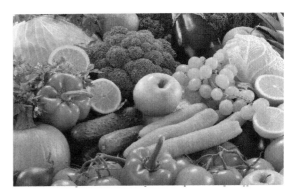

The Environmental Working Group (EWG), a non-profit organization that focuses on public health, publishes lists of produce that contain the highest concentrations of pesticide residues, also known as the dirty dozen. In 2010, the list included apples, strawberries, peaches, and blueberries.

The amount of pesticide residues on fruits and vegetables are determined based on testing done by the United States Department of Agriculture (USDA) after produce is washed with a high-power pressure water system. The dirty dozen typically contain 47 to 67 pesticides per serving—levels deemed safe by the Environmental Protection Agency (EPA). The EWG suggests that buying the organic version of the dirty dozen can reduce exposure to pesticides by 80 percent. It is important to note that the benefits of eating fresh fruits and vegetables outweigh the known risks of ingesting pesticide residues.

There are delicious and decadent healthy foods that can help your body produce beautiful skin! Here are some tips to improve your nutrition.

- Avoid and reduce synthetic products and chemicals in your food.
- Consume fewer processed and more whole foods.
- Buy products with short ingredient lists that you can understand.
- Support sustainable farming practices, buy organic and local.
- Vote with your dollar for high quality food.
- Plant a garden to provide fresh, local, organic food.

Sugar, Salt, and Fat

Sugar, salt, and fat are used as flavor enhancers to make food taste better. They are particularly effective when poor quality ingredients are used during food processing. With time, you get used to the flavor enhancers and lose the ability to taste the subtle flavors of the food itself. This means that you may eat more sugar, salt, or fat than is good for you or your skin.

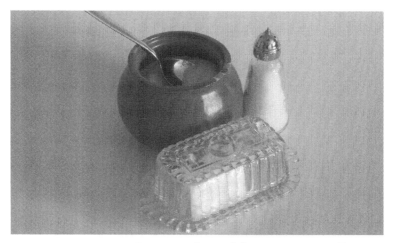

Sugar, salt and fat

As much as you may love sugar, the healthiest way to eat it is in moderation as a treat or by using sweet ingredients that contain beneficial nutrients and are metabolized more slowly by your body. Processed sugar is a simple carbohydrate that contributes empty calories and does not provide nutrients. Reducing the amount of sugar that you consume is better for your overall health and will promote beautiful skin!

When your body has to process large amounts of simple sugars, your internal organs have to work harder, resulting in unnecessary stress. Simple sugars create inflammation in the body on a cellular level, which promotes free radical production. Sugar also raises the acidity in the body potentially creating an environment for disease. Good health requires an acid alkaline balance to promote normal body function. When excess acids have to be neutralized, alkaline reserves are depleted and this leaves the body in a weakened state.

The glycemic index (GI) measures how quickly blood sugar levels rise after eating a particular type of food. It's best to eat foods that have a low glycemic index and therefore do not spike your blood sugar, and avoid processed and refined grains, which have a high GI, because they are quickly broken down by the body into sugar. These foods include refined sugar, white bread, white rice, white pasta, and white flour pastries.

To reduce the amount of simple sugars that are ingested, substitute sweeteners with lower GIs like coconut palm sugar or dried dates. To reduce simple sugars in baked goods, use whole grain flour or buy products made with whole grains. With time, your taste buds will adjust and you will enjoy eating less sweet, more complex foods that are healthier for you.

Over-consumption of salt forces the kidneys to hold more water to maintain the body's chemical balance between sodium, potassium, and water. The extra stored water raises blood pressure and puts stress on the kidneys, arteries, heart, and brain. As with sugars, with time, your taste buds may be retrained by gradually reducing the amount of salt consumed. Taste your food before adding salt; reduce the amount of salt added to your meal, and cook without salt. Compared to whole foods, processed foods typically contain large amounts of sodium. If you do eat processed food, try to select brands with reduced sodium content.

Fats are nutrients that give you energy and help the body absorb the fat-soluble vitamins A, D, E, and K. Fats are either saturated or unsaturated, and most foods with fat have both types. But usually there is more of one kind of fat than the other.

Saturated fats are solid at room temperature and found in animal foods, such as milk, cheese, and meat. They are also found in tropical oils such as coconut oil, palm oil, cocoa butter and hydrogenated fats, which are synthetically produced by adding hydrogen, heat and pressure. Adding hydrogen saturates a fat and produces trans fatty acids, which have been associated with an increased risk of heart disease. Hydrogenated trans fats have been used extensively in foods, including:

- processed foods
- snack foods, such as chips and crackers
- cookies
- some margarine and salad dressings
- foods made with partially hydrogenated oils

In recent years, the dangers of trans fats have become widely known prompting many companies to minimize or eliminate its use. Likewise, you should eat as little trans fat as possible.

Unsaturated fat, mostly found in plants, is liquid at room temperature. Monounsaturated fat and polyunsaturated fat are types of unsaturated fat. Monounsaturated fat is found in canola, olive, and peanut oils. Eating foods that are high in monounsaturated fats may help lower your "bad" (LDL) cholesterol and help to keep "good" (HDL) cholesterol levels high and lower your risk of heart disease.

Polyunsaturated fat is mainly found in safflower, sunflower, sesame, soybean, and corn oils. Polyunsaturated fat is also the main fat found in seafood. Eating polyunsaturated fat in place of saturated fat may also lower LDL cholesterol. Omega-3 is found in fish, one reason nutritionists recommend eating fish at least once a week and consuming 250 mg of these omega-3 fatty acids daily.

The medical community's attitude towards fats continues to evolve. While it is common knowledge that unsaturated fats are beneficial on many levels, recent information has indicated that saturated fats may have more benefits than previously thought. For example, it has been found that enzymes convert saturated animal fat into a monounsaturated fat, which is easier to metabolize. This finding may make consumption of animal fats healthier than previously thought.

Another example is coconut oil, a plant-based saturated fat that may have excellent health benefits despite past perceptions. In the 1980s, coconut oil got a bad rap because it is a saturated fat. The vegetable oil industry initiated a negative ad campaign criticizing tropical oils. As a result tropical oils fell out of favor and hydrogenated vegetable oils—high in trans fatty acids—replaced them. Tests to assess the health impacts of coconut oil were conducted on hydrogenated coconut oil, which showed that hydrogenated coconut oil is unhealthy. Any hydrogenated oil is unhealthy! However, tests were not conducted on unrefined, raw, organic coconut oil. Today, experts look at populations who consume raw coconut oil and find them to have low rates of heart disease.

Coconut oil is a saturated fat made up of medium- and short-chain fatty acids (MCFAs and SCFAs), which the body converts to energy instead of storing as fat. MCFAs help protect against heart disease and have many other health benefits. The MCFAs in coconut oil contain lauric acid, caprylic acid, and capric acid, which are beneficial to your health when consumed. Raw organic coconut oil is being used extensively for cooking and personal care products in health food communities with many praises for taste and health benefits.

Fat-soluble toxins can accumulate and may be stored in your body fat. Practice caution with your health and focus on consuming organic fats regardless of the type of fat that is used.

Whole Grains

There is controversy in the nutrition world about whether folks should include grains in their diet. If you are curious about this, observe how many of your calories come from grains and baked goods compared to the calories that you derive from proteins, seeds, vegetables, and fruit. Try replacing grains with vegetables and protein and see how you feel.

The concept behind eliminating grains from the diet is based on evolution. Modern humans evolved for approximately 200,000 years as hunters and gatherers without grains. When agriculture developed around 10,000 BC, diets started including baked goods and grains. In addition, many believe the wheat flour available today, is "not your grandmothers wheat" due to genetic engineering.

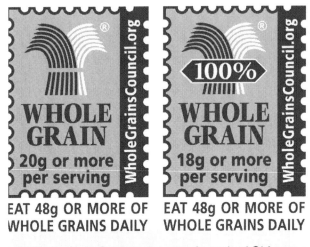

® Whole Grain Stamps are a trademark of Oldways
Preservation Trust and the Whole Grains Council,
www.wholegrainscouncil.org

You may be aware of these issues due to the recent availability of gluten-free food products for people who have Celiac disease and are allergic to wheat. If you do eat grains, avoid simple carbohydrates including white rice and white flour, which rapidly convert into simple sugars in your body and raise blood sugar levels. If you are allergic to wheat, you can use flour that is made from other sources such as coconut or quinoa flour.

Replace processed refined grains in your diet at every opportunity with whole grains, which are rich in vitamins and fiber. Look for the words *whole wheat* on ingredient lists. If it only says *wheat* it is not the whole grain and is essentially the same as refined white flour. You can also look for the Whole Grain Council's stamp on the package.

The healthiest bread and tortillas are made from organic sprouted whole grains. It may take time to adjust your taste buds to eating sprouted whole grain products if you are used to eating refined grain products. Organic sprouted grain breads were primarily available from health food stores but are becoming more available. The next best bread would be that made with organic whole grains.

Try to convert from refined grain to whole grain products. It will be worth the transition because the calories that you consume will be more nutrient rich.

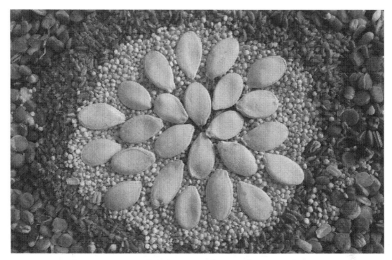

Grains and seeds

HYDRATION

Non-water beverages are popular in our culture. These beverages are often loaded with sugar, synthetic chemicals, and calories. Advertising and media promote the consumption of sodas, energy drinks, and sweet coffee drinks which contain ingredients that do not promote beautiful skin. Fruit juices contain concentrated sugars that can raise your blood sugar to unhealthy levels. It's best to eat the whole fruit to slow down digestion of fruit sugars. Wean yourself from sweet drinks and with time, your taste buds will change and you'll begin to appreciate a glass of water.

Some beverages that are good for your skin include green tea (unsweetened); green smoothies consisting of fruit mixed with a handful of spinach or kale to provide a variety of nutrients and fiber; vegetable juicing helps to make your body more alkaline and provides concentrated nutrients that are easily absorbed into the bloodstream because the fiber is removed.

Kombucha, a fermented, naturally carbonated, beverage, has recently become available in health food stores. The drink dates back to second century BC China where it was referred to as the *tea of immortality*. You can also easily make kombucha at home, using recipes found on the Internet.

Kombucha can taste sweet, although it has only two grams of sugar. To some it tastes vinegary. Kombucha begins as a mixture of tea and sugar that is digested and fermented—its alcohol content is less than three percent—into a healthful elixir via a symbiotic relationship between bacteria and yeast. Kombucha contains enzymes, probiotics, antioxidants, and vitamins including folic acid, other B vitamins, gluconic acid, amino acids, and Vitamin C.

Kombucha drinkers report many healing properties. However, it should be noted that currently available scientific evidence does not support these claims. Serious side effects and occasional deaths have been linked with drinking Kombucha tea, which can be contaminated with molds or fungus if not properly fermented. Kombucha is easy to make and only requires sanitary kitchen practices to be successful.

NUTRACEUTICALS

The term nutraceutical is derived from the words nutrition and pharmaceutical and applies to a range of products that are considered to promote health and provide protection against disease. Nutraceuticals may be supplements that consist of herbs, vitamins, minerals and more. When integrated into a healthy lifestyle, these supplements may be beneficial and promote good health. There are many choices available, based on your needs. Nutraceuticals are used to supplement healthy eating and promote healthy skin. Adding nutraceuticals to your diet should be a personal choice based on specific health requirements and goals. To learn more about nutraceuticals and to make appropriate choices, educate yourself before integrating supplements into your lifestyle.

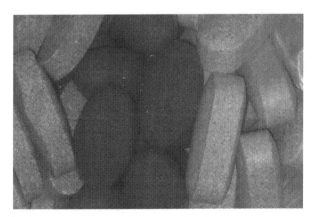

Nutraceuticals

EXERCISE

If you are not accustomed to exercising regularly, start a program to integrate physical movement into your life. Begin slowly and do what feels comfortable. At a minimum, move your body regularly. Try different types of exercises that you can integrate into your routine including yoga, strength training, and cardiovascular activities. Cross training or doing a variety of different exercises is the best method for improving overall endurance, strength, balance, and flexibility. Integrating exercise into play improves your overall quality of life.

Always check with your physician before beginning a new exercise routine. Try to find seamless ways to integrate more exercise into your life such as walking or biking for errands instead of using the car; this provides an efficient, environmental, economical, and healthy way to promote good circulation and benefit your skin! Promote family exercise and enjoy time together while doing something fun and healthy. Get in a half hour to an hour of cardio exercise six days a week to get the full potential out of your exercise routine. Exercise at a gym, at home, and in your neighborhood to create the most flexible exercise program possible.

You do not need to do hardcore, rigorous exercise to experience the benefits that exercise has to offer. A great program might include daily walking, training with weights, or working against your own weight by doing push-ups and pull ups. You might even choose to challenge yourself once or twice a week by sprinting and integrating exercises that increase flexibility and balance.

Exercise provides many benefits including:

- increased circulation
- increased metabolism
- strengthened lung capacity
- strengthened heart function
- strengthened immune system
- improved mood
- weight loss and maintenance
- increased muscle strength
- improved brain function
- better sleep
- better sex
- stress reduction
- etc., etc., etc.!

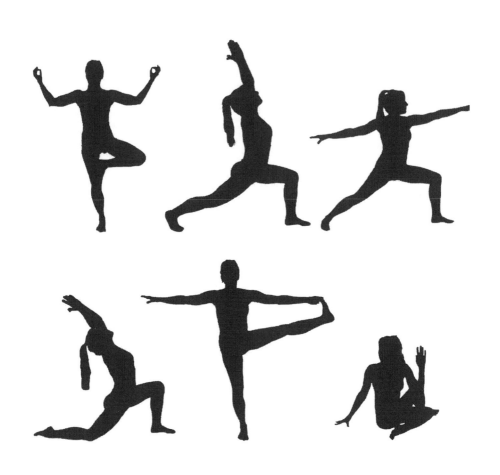

Yoga poses

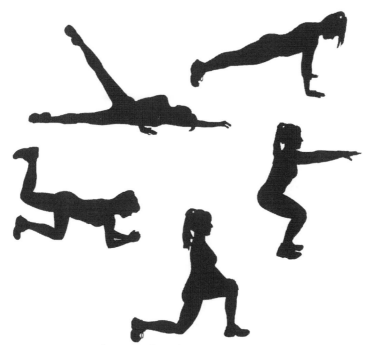

Strengthening exercises

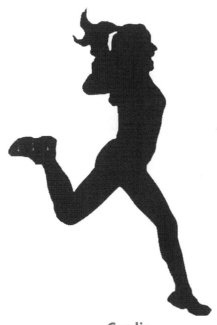

Cardio

REST

How great is a good night's rest? It is beneficial to your body and mind and is terrific for your skin. Practice good sleep hygiene by incorporating some quiet time into your routine before you go to sleep. Visualize images that are peaceful to you. This will help you to relax and wind down before laying your head on your pillow to enter into slumber land.

Seek ways to support a good sleep habit for your health and for your skin.

MENTAL ATTITUDE

Your mental attitude can affect your health. Think about a time when you heard bad news. Did you experience a physical reaction to the news? Did you get a headache, an upset stomach, or a stiff neck? Now think about a happy time. Did you feel elation, comfort, contentment, or maybe get more energy?

Stress causes the body to produce the hormones cortisol and epinephrine. Cortisol raises blood sugar levels, causes collagen to become rigid, and increases facial lines and wrinkles. Epinephrine decreases blood flow, circulation, delivery of oxygen and nutrients, and increases the presence of toxins in the skin, resulting in a dull complexion. To avoid this, try to decrease the amount of stress in your life through daily exercise, yoga, meditation and other methods to manage stress and reduce cortisol production.

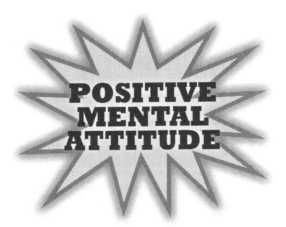

Life is full of wonderful people, mean people, and sometimes wonderful people are mean. While it is always better to avoid emotionally unhealthy or selfish people who hurt others, sometimes life doesn't give you a choice. That is why it is important to focus on the good to maintain a healthy mental state.

One way to improve your mood and promote happiness is by keeping a slight smile on your face throughout the day. This simple exercise not only changes your brain chemistry but also proves that even a fake smile can make you feel good!

Tip: Start by integrating small changes into your routine; it takes three weeks to make a habit:

- **Take a daily walk. Work up to an hour of exercise most days.**
- **Exercise to keep your brain strong.**
- **Replace a short car trip with a walk.**
- **Eat more vegetable and fruits; eat nutrient rich super foods.**
- **Eliminate soda and sweetened drinks from your diet.**
- **Drink water; flavor it with cucumber or lemon slices.**
- **Drink fresh green juice on an empty stomach.**
- **Use a refillable bottle to monitor your water intake.**
- **Take beginner's yoga or a stretching class.**
- **Nurture a soothing bedtime environment.**
- **Take a risk; try something new to keep your brain healthy.**
- **Think of solutions.**
- **Surround yourself with inclusive, positive, and kind people.**
- **Practice wearing a slight smile throughout the day.**
- **Be grateful.**

OIL CLEANSING METHOD

Skin care products, lack of good hygiene, and other reasons can cause the skin's natural oil production to go out of balance. To maintain good skin health, it is vital to wash your face each night to remove makeup, dirt, and impurities. There are many products and methods to cleanse the face, so choose a cleansing method that works for your skin type.

My preferred method is the oil cleansing method (OCM) that uses castor oil mixed with another oil of your choice. Castor oil has potent anti-inflammatory properties, is healing, and cleansing. The OCM, a wonderful facial cleanser that is easily and inexpensively made at home, works on the concept that like dissolves like. The OCM dissolves natural skin oils that have become hardened with impurities, unclogs pores, eliminates blackheads, and removes peeling skin that may result from cosmetic dermatology treatments or the use of strong cosmeceuticals.

As dirt plugs are removed and unclogged pores begin to function properly, they may overproduce the skins natural oils. With time, the skin will adjust to the use of OCM and begin to function normally. The skin will also become less red and irritated as dirt and blackheads are removed.

The OCM is typically used once a day, at night, to cleanse and remove makeup, sunscreen, and the day from your face. Massage the oil blend into your face and neck for about five minutes. You may feel the small hard oil plugs that are removed from your pores as you massage. Rinse thoroughly by vigorously massaging warm water over your face and neck and rub dry with a towel. If desired, you can use a physical exfoliation method, like a microfiber facecloth or face scrubber, to remove any residual oil from the skin. After the OCM cleansing, use your normal evening skin care routine. In the morning, there is no need to use a cleanser; instead just rinse your face with water before applying your daytime skin care products. The OCM is gentle, effective, and costs pennies to make.

Tip: Use the OCM a couple times a week followed by a good scrub with a microfiber cloth. Other nights, use only the microfiber cloth to scrub every inch of your face and neck; your face will be perfectly clean. A water rinse in the morning is all you need. This routine has been a standard step in my own skincare routine for years; no longer is there any need for me to buy cleansers. In fact, my skin care routine is more enjoyable without them. Try it and see what you think.

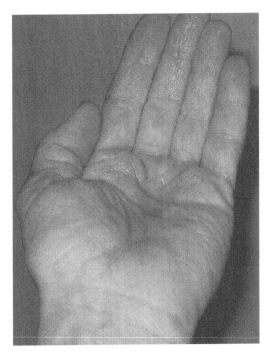

Preparing for the oil cleansing method

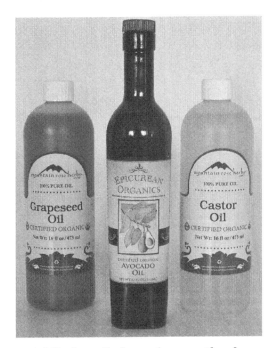

Oils for oil cleansing method

SKIN CARE PRODUCTS

Most over the counter (OTC) skin care products can be made at home. DIY skin care can range from simple to complex depending on your desire and comfort level. When you make DIY skin care products you can create and use high quality skin cleansers, moisturizers, and treatments that not only cost much less, but are also often much stronger and more effective than OTC products. DIY skin care products can be made without the undesirable additives that may be present in OTC products. The cosmetic industry is not required to test products for safety or effectiveness because they are not subject to federal regulations under Food & Drug Administration rules, therefore a large variety of ingredients may be added to cosmetics, including undesirable additives.

With the availability of pure active ingredients, DIY enthusiasts can personally design and prepare high concentration, additive-free products. The DIY skin care community often shares their experiences and their favorite skin care recipes on the Internet so that others may benefit. Blending your own skin care products can be a fun and beneficial hobby. If you read the thousands of posts that happy DIYers write about making and using their own skin care products and the great results that they experience, you will see that DIY skin care is fiercely popular among those in the know.

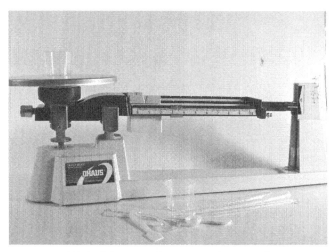

<u>Weighing and measuring tools</u>

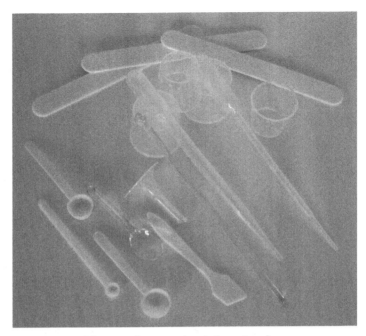

Measuring and mixing tools

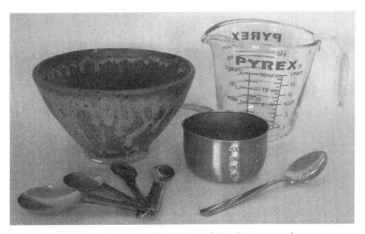

Measuring and mixing kitchen tools

There are a variety of ways to blend your own DIY skin care products and cosmeceuticals. You can add an individual cosmeceutical or active ingredient to a serum, lotion, or cream that you have at home; develop your own recipes using a combination of active ingredients; or find recipes on the Internet for your particular skin care needs. It is even possible to find recipes for popular OTC products and duplicate them at home for a fraction of the cost.

When blending your own skin care products you may:

- use specific active ingredients
- use high concentrations of active ingredients
- save money
- avoid synthetic fillers
- develop high quality customized skin care systems

For example, a well-formulated, top quality, high concentration, vitamin C serum can cost $80 or more for one ounce in retail outlets. This same serum may be made at home for a few dollars an ounce. Vitamin C serum is extremely beneficial and is typically used daily in the morning.

Active ingredients may be blended to make personalized, high concentration toners, serums, lotions, and creams. These products have unique properties that make them useful for different skin care needs.

TONER

A toner is a liquid with astringent properties that may be used to shrink or constrict tissues. It is also used to further clean the skin after washing, to exfoliate dead skin cells, and to refine pores. It is typically used after washing the face and before applying other skin care products.

SERUM

A serum is a thick liquid that penetrates the skin deeper than a cream because of high concentrations of active ingredients, smaller molecules, and a watery base. Serums deposit nutrients in the skin and are tailored for specific skin care concerns such as hyperpigmentation, anti-aging, or brightening the complexion.

Serums should be applied after washing the face and applying toner, but before applying moisturizer. After applying the serum, you should wait five to 10 minutes before applying moisturizer to allow the active ingredients in the serum to penetrate. A serum may or may not be moisturizing, depending on the ingredients.

LOTION

A lotion is a liquid moisturizer that is lighter than a cream moisturizer. It does not penetrate into deeper layers of the skin but instead deposits moisturizing components on the outermost layers of skin. Lotion is beneficial for those with oily skin or those who do not need a heavy moisturizer.

CREAM

A cream is a heavy moisturizer useful for dry skin. A cream does not penetrate into the deeper layers of the skin but deposits moisturizers on the surface of the skin.

TREATMENT AREAS

We all know that skin care products and treatments are applied to the face. But to further support firm, healthy skin it is important to also apply skin care products and treatments to the front and back of the neck, behind the ears, on the chest, and on the hands.

The neck and chest skin is delicate so if exposed to the elements without adequate protection and nourishment, it will ultimately show signs of aging and begin to sag. If the skin on the front and back of the neck and behind the ears is protected and nourished, it will remain firm, maintain elasticity, minimize sag, and support the appearance of the facial skin. Every little bit helps!

The chest area is easily exposed to the sun as a result of low neckline clothing. Over time, exposed and undernourished chest skin will show signs of sun damage, including age spots and a loss of skin elasticity. The chest skin can remain firm and unblemished if skin care products and sun protection are used regularly.

Age spots on the hands can be prevented by applying skin care products and by protecting the hands from the sun.

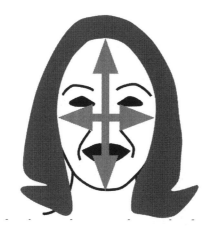

Apply products to the entire face and behind the ears

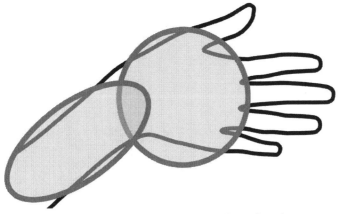

Apply products to the hand and wrist

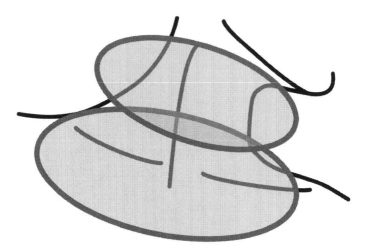

Apply products to the neck and chest

You can economically use high quality skin care products all over your body. After applying premium cosmeceutical skin care products to your face and neck and before wiping the residue off of your hands, place a few drops of water in the palms of your hands to dilute the product residue and apply the thinned product to your hands, chest, arms, and legs.

Tip: Make your own skin care products and use the highest quality ingredients at a reasonable cost. My two favorite serums cost only a few dollars an ounce to make and they are extremely effective. You only need a couple of cosmeceutical ingredients to make a strong, safe and effective skin care product.

SKIN PENETRATION

The stratum corneum, or horny layer of the epidermis, provides a protective barrier that retains moisture and prevents unwanted substances from entering the body. This protective barrier also makes it challenging for the epidermis to absorb cosmeceutical products to promote the biologic processes that produce new collagen. Laboratory tests show that water soluble products can enter the skin one thousand times faster than when the stratum corneum is not present.

SKIN PATHWAYS

Skin care products penetrate the skin through different paths. The appendageal route allows products to pass through the stratum corneum via sweat glands or hair follicles. This route is considered a minor route for the penetration of ions and large molecules.

The intercellular route allows products to penetrate the stratum corneum by moving in between skin cells. Fat loving molecules use the intercellular route.

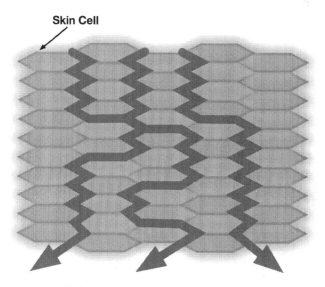

Intercellular route for product penetration

The transcellular, or intracellular, route allows products to penetrate by moving through skin cells. Water-loving molecules use the intracellular route, which is considered the primary route and barrier to product penetration.

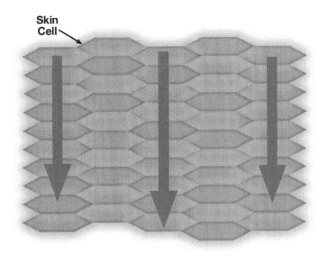

Transcellular route for product penetration

INCREASING PRODUCT PENETRATION

Chemical skin treatments may be used to increase the penetration of actives through the skin. Penetration of skin care products may be increased when supersaturated or high concentrations of active ingredients are used. These micro-emulsions form a chemical concentration gradient that moves the skin care product across the skin barrier and enhances penetration of cosmeceuticals into the skin.

Specially formulated skin care products use extremely small particles to transport active ingredients through the stratum corneum. They include formulations referred to as "liposomes, nanoemulsions, and solid-lipid nanoparticles." Other special formulations are transferosomes that are able to squeeze through tiny skin pores.

Hydrated skin increases penetration. When products deliver water or hold water in the skin, the horny layer opens up, allowing for better penetration of active ingredients.

Chemical enhancers, such as solvents like alcohol, may be used to increase product penetration. Chemical enhancers include products that remove lipids from the stratum corneum, displace water, or loosen the structure of the stratum corneum.

However, use of chemical enhancers may irritate the skin.

Physical skin treatments that may be used to increase the penetration of actives through the skin include:

- Phonophoresis (sonoporesis) uses ultrasound energy to enlarge intercellular routes, disrupt lipids, and increase the movement of active molecules through the skin.

- Iontophoresis uses a device that generates a low electric current that has the same charge as the active skin care product that is applied. The current repels the active product and pushes it into the skin.

- Electro-osmosis creates an electric field that increases skin penetration and carries dissolved actives into the skin.

- Electroporation uses a higher electric voltage over a short time interval to enhance penetration of active ingredients into the skin. The higher voltage results in a brief opening of water pores in the skin.

- Diffusion, eletrophoresis, and electro-osmosis are used to enhance penetration of molecules through the pores.

A recently developed, highly effective method to increase product penetration uses micro-needles, also known as dermarollers. The tiny needles are used to poke channels through the stratum corneum. The channels increase the permeability of the skin and allow active molecules to penetrate. When combined with microelectronic devices, product penetration can be maximized.

To get the maximum effect from your high quality skin care products, use several methods to increase the penetration of active ingredients through the skin barrier such as integrating passive (chemical) and active (physical) product penetration treatments into your skin care routine.

....

Tip: Product penetration is important. When you use high quality ingredients, maximize their effectiveness by preparing your skin for application. Foremost, exfoliate dead skins cells regularly and pick a device to enhance product penetration that fits your preference and lifestyle.

ACTIVE INGREDIENTS

Almost any active ingredient that is available in OTC products may be purchased for DIY skin care formulations including vitamins, nutrients, antioxidants, peptides, collagen, and acids.

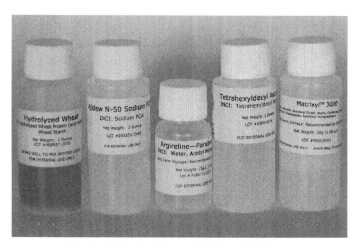

Active ingredients in liquid form

Currently, cosmeceuticals and other active ingredients are primarily purchased from Internet stores. New resources for active ingredients are becoming available as the DIY skin care industry grows. Internet sites that sell active ingredients usually provide information describing their properties and include instructions for proper use. At a minimum, usage and storage instructions will be provided on the website and/or with the shipping materials.

There are hundreds of ingredients available for making DIY skin care products. A few popular options are described in the following text to provide examples of the variety of products that are available and their uses. If you would like more information about the active ingredients listed below or other active ingredients, visit DIY skin care Internet stores to view product lists and descriptions or research journal articles for information or studies on active ingredients.

Cosmeceuticals, or active ingredients, are categorized as antioxidants, anti-inflammatories, collagen promoting, growth factors, peptides, neurotransmitters, acids and enzymes, skin lightening, carrier and essential oils, and herbal tinctures.

Always use active ingredients at the recommended concentrations and test your specially blended skin care products on a small patch of skin to check for potential allergic reactions prior to applying mixtures to your face.

Before formulating a new product with multiple active ingredients, making a new recipe, or combining products with different active ingredients, search Internet skin care sites to identify the best use based on your combination of active ingredients. For example, it is generally recommended that retinoids be used at night as opposed to the morning because your skin becomes sensitive to UV rays and the sun may deactivate the retinoid.

Another example is that of avoiding the use of glycolic acid serum or moisturizer at the same time that hydroquinone, vitamin C serum, or a retinoid are used because they can be deactivated by the glycolic acid. Depending on the concentrations, each of these active ingredients may be irritating and may over-irritate the skin if used together, aside from interacting with each other.

Typically, people will alternate use of an individual active ingredient throughout the day. For example, one will use retinoids at night and vitamin C serum in the morning.

ANTIOXIDANTS

It is widely accepted that aging is associated with free radical damage. Antioxidants prevent oxidative damage while neutralizing free radicals, help reduce inflammation, and reduce oxidative cell damage. As we age, naturally occurring antioxidant levels in the skin decrease. Providing the skin with antioxidant, anti-inflammatory nourishment is a major part of minimizing and reducing the rate at which the skin ages.

There are many antioxidants that help reduce free radicals, prevent skin damage, repair damaged skin, and provide anti-inflammatory benefits including Coenzyme Q10 and green tea with polyphenols.

Using a blend of several antioxidants can be more effective than using a single antioxidant. For example, recent studies have shown that a blend of niacinamide and NAG (*N*-acetyl glucosamine) can be effective in reducing melanin production and diminish the appearance of hyperpigmentation.

Here is a brief summary of select popular antioxidants and anti-inflammatory ingredients that may be found in cosmeceuticals:

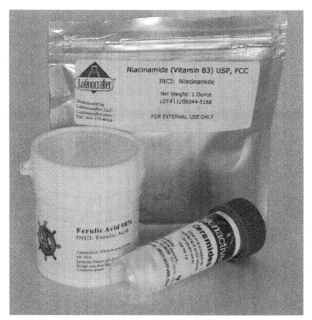

Active ingredients in powder form

Aloe vera is an effective anti-inflammatory. Aloe vera is considered to be biologically active with over 75 potentially active constituents that promote wound healing and enhance collagen production. The plant may be used directly on the skin. Break off an aloe vera leaf, wash it, cut off the edges, slice the leaf in half to expose the gelatinous interior and rub it directly on the skin to heal and soothe.

Alpha lipoic acid (ALA) is a potent antioxidant that inhibits wrinkling by fighting free radicals. It has been found to increase the effects of skin rejuvenation during cosmetic dermatology treatments.

Co-enzyme Q-10, also known as ubiquinone, is an effective antioxidant and an important element in cell respiration. Topical application stimulates cell processes and promotes production of new collagen. Idebenone is sold as a synthetic form of Coenzyme Q10. Idebenone has a different structure and may cause allergic reactions.

Dimethylethanolamine (DMAE) is a powerful antioxidant that stimulates nerve and muscle function. DMAE contracts muscles and can prevent and reverse skin sagging.

Ferulic acid (FA) is a strong antioxidant with a wide range of beneficial actions against disease. This strong skin cell membrane antioxidant scavenges free radicals, making it a terrific ingredient in DIY skin care products. FA is reported to decrease inflammatory processes and reduce the impact of UV radiation, thus protecting the skin from photo damage. Use of FA in a 15 percent solution with L-ascorbic acid and 1 percent vitamin E improves the stability of the L-ascorbic acid and increases skin protection from UV exposure.

Glucosamine (n-acetyl glucosamine or NAG) inhibits the production of melanin and hyperpigmentation. It has antioxidant and anti-inflammatory properties and promotes the production of hyaluronic acid, which is hydrating. NAG also promotes collagen production.

Grape seed extract has been shown to be beneficial during wound healing. It provides protection against photo damage and increases the absorption of other vitamins.

Green tea is a strong antioxidant. It contains epigallocatechin gallate (ECCG), a catechin or antioxidant with strong anti-inflammatory properties for skin. The antioxidants in green tea fight free radicals and inflammation.

Hyaluronic acid (HA) has a large capacity to hold water and helps keep skin moist. HA helps to maintain thickness in the dermis and supports connective tissue.

Isoflavones are plant estrogens that are found in soybeans. They are referred to as flavonoids or phytochemicals and are natural plant components. One form of isoflavone, Genistein, has been shown to promote collagen production. Skin benefits that are derived from the use of isoflavones may be due to the presence of plant estrogens.

Methylsulfonylmethane (MSM) is a sulfur compound that is a vital component of skin cells. MSM helps to maintain the flexibility and elasticity of body tissue and maintains membrane permeability. MSM promotes soft moisturized skin making it an important ingredient in a skin care program.

Niacinamide has been shown to promote synthesis of fats, collagen production and anti-inflammatory benefits. It also inhibits the production of melanin.

Resveratrol is an antioxidant found in grapes. Initial studies have shown that resveratrol antioxidants protect against free radicals and promote healing of skin disorders.

Retinoic acid, marketed as Tretinoin and Retin-A, when used at concentrations between 0.05 and 0.1 percent, can reverse photo-aging and improve the appearance of wrinkles by promoting healing and collagen production. The skin can immediately use retinoic acid. Retinoids have a high concentration of retinoic acid and may cause irritation, redness, dryness, and peeling until the skin becomes accustomed to them. Clinical studies have shown that retinoic acid reduces the signs of aging by decreasing melanin production, reducing the depth of wrinkles, increasing collagen production, and smoothing the stratum corneum. Retin-A is available only by prescription in the United States. Insurance does not cover its usage for mature skin care and one tube may cost $40 to $75. Retin-A may be purchased in Mexico without a prescription. It may also be purchased from overseas pharmacies without a prescription at a reduced price, although some sites require that you provide your primary healthcare providers contact information. Ordering Retin-A from an overseas pharmacy, a half dozen tubes per order, allows me to realize large cost savings.

Retinol, retinaldehyde, and retinyl palmitate are less irritating, slower acting, do not require a prescription, and are less expensive than retinoic acid. The body needs to convert these forms into retinoic acid to be useable; this results in a lower concentration of retinoic acid available to the skin. Depending on the strength and the length of time used, retinols can be effective in treating photo-aging by promoting normal growth of the rete ridge, and enhancing oxygen and nutrient nourishment to the epidermis.

Sea kelp bioferment is a nutritional active that contains cellular components from algae. It is derived from fermented sea kelp and has a thin gel consistency. It is used as an oil free emollient base and can increase moisture by creating a protective film.

Vitamin A plays an important role in the production of collagen and is degraded by sun exposure. It comes in several forms such as retinoic acid or retinol. Retinoic acid and retinoids cause sun sensitivity, so it is best to use them at night and to use sunscreen daily.

Vitamin C serum has proven effective in skin care maintenance and can be used daily for optimum benefits. Vitamin C is one of the most studied skin care antioxidants. As we age, vitamin C concentrations in the skin decrease. Use of vitamin C in cosmeceuticals has been shown to thicken skin and to reduce fine wrinkling. In addition, vitamin C provides protection against sun damage by neutralizing free radicals generated by sun exposure.

Vitamin C is essential for biochemical functions, helps to maintain a strong immune response, supports vitamin E regeneration, helps to heal wounds, promotes production of collagen and elastin, and helps to repair the rete ridge promoting development of new blood vessels and thereby increasing nourishment to the epidermis.

Vitamin C is available in several forms, including: L-ascorbic acid (LAA, water soluble), tetrahexyldecyl ascorbate (oil soluble), and magnesium ascorbyl phosphate (MAP)—skin enzymes convert MAP into ascorbic acid.

Tetrahexyldecyl ascorbate is nonirritating and may be used in an oil-based serum. MAP is water soluble, stable, and mild and may be used by those who cannot tolerate LAA. Appendix D contains a recipe for a lovely, high-concentration DIY vitamin C serum that can be made for a fraction of the cost of retail versions.

Vitamin E is oil soluble. It consists of eight different forms:

- Alpha, beta, gamma, and delta tocopherol;
- Alpha, beta, gamma, and delta tocotrienol.

Alpha tocopherol is the most active in humans. Vitamin E is available in its natural form (labeled with a *d*) or as a synthetic product (labeled with a *dl*). Vitamin E has been found to protect cell membranes by reducing free radicals and protecting the skin from sun damage. It has also been shown that d-alpha tocopherol, in a 2 to 5 percent concentration, is effective in improving the quality of the skin.

Each form of vitamin E has a unique function; much of the past research focused on the effectiveness of the tocopherols. However, recent studies show that tocotrienols provide strong neuroprotective and antioxidant functions that are different from the tocopherol functions.

Zinc is an effective antioxidant that provides protection from the sun as a physical sunblock, plays an important role in wound healing, and has been shown to act as a skin lightening ingredient.

GROWTH FACTORS

Growth factors are large molecules that require special delivery methods to allow them to penetrate through the stratum corneum. When the skin is injured, the body naturally concentrates growth factors at the site of the wound to promote collagen production and to repair photo-damaged skin. A trial study showed that when synthetic growth factors were applied to the skin, they accelerated wound healing and stimulated collagen production. After 60 days, there was a 37 percent increase in new collagen and a 27 percent increase in the thickness of the epidermis.

Epidermal growth factor (EGF) is a small protein that carries growth messages and is released by cells during wound healing. EGF is important in the regulation of cell development. It binds to cell receptors and initiates a cascade of biochemical reactions that increase energy production and protein synthesis.

Keratinocyte growth factor (KGF) increases cell growth in the skin and erases wrinkles by enhancing facial volume and plumping skin cells. KGF is reported to help cells multiply up to eight times faster than normal. The human body produces growth factors naturally to heal wounds, but clinical studies have shown that artificial KGF, when applied topically, can make second-degree burns heal faster. The binding of the growth factor to receptors on cell membranes initiates a cascade of molecular events that eventually leads to cell division.

Furfuryladenine (kinetin) is a growth factor that is derived from plants and has been shown to decrease and delay age-related changes to the skin. A 0.05 percent concentration has been shown to decrease wrinkling by 13 percent, hyperpigmentation by 27 percent, and roughness by 60 percent when applied twice a day over a period of 24 weeks.

PEPTIDES

The skin is made up of collagen, which is made up of proteins. Proteins are long chains of amino acids. Shorter segments of proteins are referred to as peptides and are biochemically active in the skin.

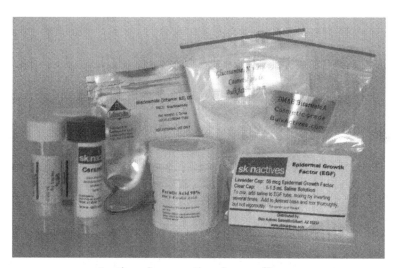

Anti-aging, active ingredients

Peptides have been shown to stimulate collagen production in the dermis during wound healing. When peptides are combined they can stimulate skin repair or slow down skin aging processes. Studies show that application of peptides over a period of four to eight weeks results in significant improvement in the skins appearance. Peptides are separated into three different categories: signal, carrier, and neurotransmitter-inhibiting.

Signal peptides may promote stimulation of collagen and improved skin conditions. Palmitoyl pentapeptide (matrixyl) is a signal peptide.

Carrier peptides are small and may be used to deliver active ingredients because they are able to penetrate into deeper, biologically-active, layers of the skin. Copper peptide is a carrier peptide.

Neuropeptides, when applied topically, may penetrate into the muscle and block nerve signals decreasing muscle contraction and reducing the appearance of wrinkles. Gamma amino butyric acid (GABA) and argireline are neuropeptides. They are used in skin care to lessen the effects of wrinkles as part of an anti-aging regimen. If they are able to penetrate muscle they may also reduce muscle contractions much like Botox, however, clinical studies have not been conducted to support this claim.

NEUROTRANSMITTERS

Amino acids or peptides break down into neurotransmitters or signaling molecules that send chemical messages or signals between cells.

DMAE (dimethylaminoethanol) is believed to increase neurotransmitter messenger signals that help firm skin and contract muscles. A study using a 3 percent concentration over a period of 18 weeks showed improvement in wrinkles, sagging neck skin, and circles around the eyes.

ACIDS AND ENZYMES

Chemical peels are used to exfoliate the outermost layer of the skin by chemically removing dead skin cells with acids of varying strengths or enzymes. Common acids include alpha hydroxy acids (AHAs), beta hydroxy acids (BHAs), tetrachloroethylene (TCA), and Jessner's peel. Enzymes include: pumpkin, papaya, and pineapple extracts. Peels result in a brighter and fresher looking complexion and help reduce the appearance of hyperpigmentation.

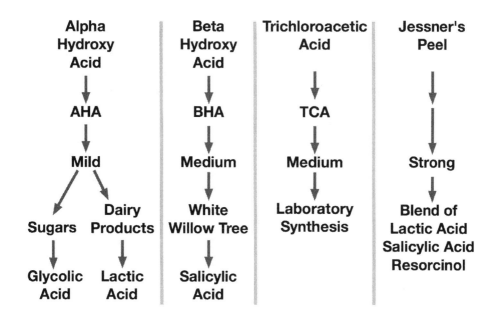

Facial acids

Acids

Alpha hydroxy acids (AHA) are water-soluble and include citric, glycolic, and lactic acids. DIY application of AHAs are used at concentrations between 10 percent (with a pH of 3.5 or greater) and by specialists at concentrations up to 80 percent (with a pH of 3.0 or greater). AHAs are more effective at a low pH, although they can be irritating. AHA facials encourage new skin cell growth by reducing the thickness of the stratum corneum and by promoting the production of collagen and elastin.

Glycolic acid is a low to medium strength AHA that is derived from sugar cane. Glycolic acid is one of the most effective AHAs, although it is not known exactly how it works in the skin. It restores a fresh, glowing complexion, reduces skin discoloration, improves the appearance of fine lines, minimizes the appearance of pores, unplugs oil glands, increases penetration of other treatments, moisturizes, and can bleach skin discoloration. Glycolic acid penetrates the epidermis.

Lactic acid is a mild AHA acid that is derived from dairy products. For example, yogurt contains a weak strength of lactic acid and can be used as a facial mask to freshen the appearance of the skin. Pure lactic acid may be purchased for home use. Lactic acid treatments have been shown to increase the thickness of the epidermis and to smooth and reduce the thickness of the stratum corneum. Lactic acid penetrates the epidermis.

Beta hydroxy acids (BHAs) are oil soluble and can penetrate facial oils to deep clean pores. They are anti-inflammatory, antibacterial, and can be tolerated by those with rosacea.

Salicylic acid is a BHA that is able to enter the skin via hair follicles, and is widely used in OTC solutions that unplug pores, prevent acne, and reduce blackheads. This acid only penetrates the surface of the epidermis.

Trichloracetic acid (TCA) peels are synthetically-made, medium strength peels that are typically administered by a dermatologist. It is possible to safely give yourself a DIY TCA peel; however, extreme caution must be used to avoid damaging your skin. TCA peels are effective in smoothing the skin, reducing hyperpigmentation and fine lines and removing sun damaged skin. TCA solution may be purchased from Internet stores. A TCA peel penetrates the epidermis and the upper layers of the dermis.

Jessner's peel is a medium strength peel. It is a blend of salicylic acid, lactic acid, and resorcinol. Resorcinol helps remove the horny layer of the epidermis and works as an antiseptic and disinfectant at 5 to 10 percent concentrations to treat chronic skin diseases. Jessner's peel is used to exfoliate the skin surface and to penetrate deep into the skin to unclog pores and rejuvenate the skin. Jessner's peel penetrates the epidermis and the upper layers of the dermis.

Enzymes

Enzyme peels are made from papain (papaya), bromelain (pineapple), or pumpkin. Enzymes gently remove dead skin cells while nourishing the skin with phytonutrients. This is a good peel for those with sensitive skin who do not tolerate acid peels well.

Peel Treatments

For better peel results, pre-treat the skin for four to six weeks with retinoic acid, retinol, and glycolic acid. When planning a DIY peel, it is imperative that you use extreme caution. Acids and enzymes can be purchased from DIY skin care Internet stores. When you buy acids, the retailer should provide detailed usage instructions;

study these carefully before using a DIY peel. It is important to test chemical and enzyme peels on a small patch of skin before using on your face. All peels can increase skin sensitivity to the sun. Following a peel, always use sun protection to prevent photo-damage and hyperpigmentation.

SKIN LIGHTENING INGREDIENTS

Skin bleaching and skin lightening products can be used to minimize and prevent the appearance of skin discolorations, also commonly referred to as sun or age spots. When using products or methods to lighten the skin, it is vital to use sun protection during the process. Skin lightening can make the skin sun sensitive and sun exposure can result in additional hyperpigmentation.

There are different products available to bleach or lighten sunspots. Hydroquinone is considered the gold standard and is available at 4 percent concentrations by prescription and 2 percent concentrations over the counter. Hydroquinone is recognized by the U.S. Food and Drug Administration as a skin bleaching agent and may be an irritant causing redness and dryness.

The optimum skin bleaching and lightening products contain a mixture of hydroquinone combined with other ingredients. However, the blend must be properly stabilized to prevent oxidation and degradation. Other lightening compounds include kojic acid, azelaic acid, tretinoin, arbutin, licorice, and vitamin C. Skin lighteners inhibit melanin production and may be less irritating than skin bleaching.

Exfoliation methods like glycolic or lactic acid peels or dermabrasion may be used to minimize or eliminate sunspots. Use a short needle dermaroller to enhance penetration of a glucosamine and niacinimide serum or of a low concentration, oil soluble vitamin A and C serum to reduce hyperpigmentation. Always test a new skin care system on a small patch of skin for 24 hours before applying to your face.

OILS

There are many oils to choose from for your skin care needs. After reading about the properties of different oils, identify those that are best suited to your skin type. The list below provides examples of oils used in skin care; however it is not comprehensive. If you have a favorite type of oil at home or you see a particular brand of oil that interests you, research it on the Internet to learn about its skin care benefits. It is best to use raw, unrefined, organic oils for your skin care, but it is not absolutely necessary. Oils are used as carrier oils, as the foundation of a blend, or as essential oils that are used by the drop for aromatherapy purposes.

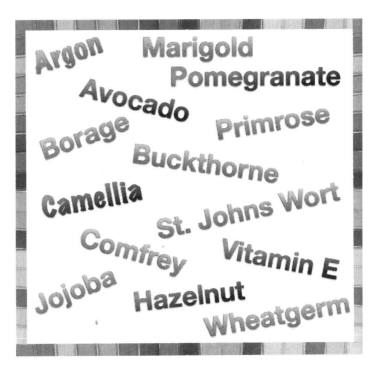

<u>Organic carrier oils</u>

Carrier Oils

Carrier oils are used as a base for cleansing, massage, and facial oils. They contain vitamins and nutrients and are used in skin care products as a source of vitamin E or for their other beneficial ingredients.

Argan oil is rich is essential fatty acids, vitamin E and more.

Avocado oil contains high concentrations of antioxidants and nutrients and is considered to be an active ingredient. One ounce of avocado oil contains 600 milligrams (mg) of vitamin A; 1,200 mg vitamin D; 9 mg vitamin E, and more. It also contains the fatty acids: linoleic, linolenic, oleic, palmitic, and palmitoleic.

Borage oil has one of the highest concentrations of gamma-linolenic acid, also known as omega-6, of the carrier oils. It is also high in salicylic acid. Borage oil has skin smoothing, anti-inflammatory and anti-septic properties.

Camellia oil is high in anti-oxidants and absorbs readily and deeply into the skin.

Castor oil has been used throughout history for its many health benefits. The thick oil is healing, cleansing, treats acne, penetrates deep layers of the skin, and has antioxidant, antibacterial, and anti-inflammatory properties. Castor oil contains essential fatty acids, which promote healthy cells. Castor oil has a softening effect on inelastic skin, nourishes dull, lifeless, dry and devitalized skin; eczema; and psoriasis.

Coconut oil is readily absorbed, lubricates, and softens the skin. It is a powerful antimicrobial with high concentrations of medium-chained fatty acids (MCFAs), which are used by the body as building blocks for tissues. One tablespoon contains seven grams of lauric acid, which has health promoting properties. Coconut oil has been used from ancient times because it is considered to have skin healing properties.

Comfrey oil has a high allantoin content, a substance that promotes new cell growth. Comfrey oil is generally used for wound healing and skin cell proliferation.

Grapeseed oil absorbs easily into the skin and does not leave a greasy feeling. Because of this, it is used as a base oil for creams, lotions, and as a general carrier oil. It has non-allergenic properties making it good for people who have sensitive skin. Grapeseed oil is a good source of vitamin E in alpha tocopherol form.

Hazelnut oil is light and easily absorbed. It is high in vitamin E and essential fatty acids and has moisturizing and anti-inflammatory properties.

Jojoba oil is a polyunsaturated liquid wax. Jojoba is good for inflamed skin, eczema, psoriasis, rough/dry skin, and acne. It penetrates the skin easily.

Olive oil is a thick and heavy oil. It contains anti-oxidants, is anti-microbial and is an excellent cleanser for dry skin.

Marigold oil has anti-bacterial, anti-fungal, and anti-oxidant properties that can calm and protect the skin.

Neem oil is exceptionally rich with a strong odor. Neem oil has moisturizing and regenerative properties.

Palm oil has a deep orange-red color due to the high concentration of beta-carotene and other carotenoids. Crude palm oil contains a high amount of vitamin E as tocotrienols, mainly consisting of gamma-tocotrienol and alpha-tocotrienol. Because of the red color, this oil is best used in a facial or in small quantities in DIY preparations.

Primrose oil is high in gamma linolenic acid and anti-inflammatory properties. This oil is used to reduce skin conditions and inflammation.

Pomegranate oil contains punicic acid, which is an omega-5 fatty acid, providing anti-oxidant properties that protect against free radicals and accelerate cellular regeneration and rejuvenation.

Rosehip oil is high in essential fatty acids, vitamin C and vitamin A and can reduce sun damage and skin discoloration.

Saint John's Wort oil has anti-viral and anti-septic properties and speeds wound healing. Its use may cause sun sensitivity.

Vitamin E oil is a heavy oil that is high in anti-oxidants. Vitamin E oil fights free radicals to reduce wrinkles and the aging process.

Wheatgerm oil is an ultra-rich oil high in anti-oxidant and regenerative properties.

Aromatherapy Oils

Aromatherapy or essential oils are aromatic, concentrated oils extracted from the flowers, fruits, bark, resins, leaves and roots of plants and trees. These oils are known for their therapeutic, cell-rejuvenating properties. It is best to use oils obtained by steam distillation or by the extraction or cold press method where the oils are squeezed from the plant materials. Oils that are extracted using solvents are referred to as absolutes or resins. Essential oils easily mix with fats and this property helps them to penetrate the skin.

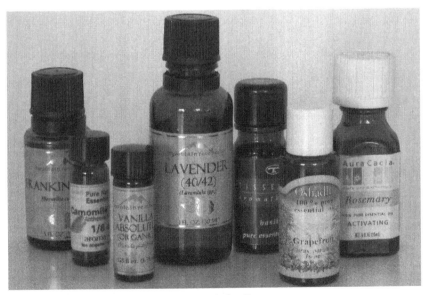

Essential oils

Please do not mistake essential oils for synthetic oils. Synthetic fragrance oils and perfumes contain a multitude of chemicals and can cause allergic reactions and weaken the immune system. Fragrances and perfumes do not have health promoting properties. Although fragrances may be present in store-bought creams, perfumes and fragrances should never be used in your DIY skin care products. Likewise, try to avoid lotions and creams made with perfumes or fragrances.

Aromatherapy oils contain high concentrations of beneficial compounds and can be used as actives in skin care products. Essential oils are easily mixed with skin care products to enhance the appearance of your skin or to treat a variety of skin ailments. Essential oils are absorbed by the skin within two hours and penetrate deeply into the tissues.

The active properties in essential oils rejuvenate the skin by regulating capillaries and restoring vitality to tissues. Essential oils help to eliminate waste and promote the production of new skin cells.

Essential oils are concentrated and should never be applied to the skin undiluted. Blend select essential oils with a carrier oil or with cleansers, toners, serums, lotions, and creams.

Pure essential oils can be purchased from health food and Internet stores. If you are going to use essential oils, it is worth buying a reference book to identify the oils that are best for your skin type.

Each essential oil has different properties and can be used to treat different skin conditions. For example, rosehip oil is high in bio-available vitamin C and other constituents, including gamma linoleic acid that promote skin regeneration and enhance skin elasticity. The high gamma linoleic acid content helps to reduce the signs of aging, especially fine lines around the eyes and mouth.

Essential Oil	General Skin	Normal Skin	Dry Skin	Oily Skin	Mature Skin	Acne	Rejuvenation
Benzoin							X
Carrot	X		X		X		
Chamomile	X						X
Clary Sage		X	X		X		
Frankincense				X	X		X
Geranium	X	X		X			X
Lavender	X	X		X		X	X
Lemon	X			X	X		
Rose				X			X
Rosemary				X			X
Ylang	X	X		X			

Essential oils and their use with different skin types

HERBS

Herbs have been used medicinally since prehistoric times. The biochemical compositions of plants are complex and have been used as medicinal active ingredients to stimulate the skin's sebaceous gland secretions, excrete wastes, and stimulate lymph flow. Herbal tinctures concentrate these beneficial constituents and may be added to skin care products to promote collagen production and improve skin elasticity.

Tinctures are prepared by soaking herbs in 95 percent ethanol or glycerin for several weeks. The herb is entirely dissolved in the liquid leaving only the woody parts of the plant, which are discarded. Herbal active ingredients may also be purchased from Internet stores. Herbs are used in bio-cellular skin care where the herbal properties are used to stimulate the skin's own healing mechanisms for therapeutic results. Descriptions of selected beneficial herbs are provided below. Try extracts of these herbs in your skin care products or research other herbs to address your particular skin care needs.

Comfrey is high in carbohydrates. It rejuvenates the skin and contains healing, soothing, and moisture retaining properties. It is used to reverse rough, damaged skin and with time can alleviate wrinkling and promote skin elasticity. Allantoin is a component of comfrey that promotes skin cell regeneration. Allantoin counteracts dryness and cracking, stimulates growth of new skin cells, and helps sensitive skin to become more resilient.

Gotu kola or Indian pennywort was historically used to heal wounds and ulcerated skin. It promotes healing and prevents development of excess scar tissue. It has been used in Ayurvedic medicine, which focuses on prevention, to help retard the aging process. Gotu kola's active ingredients promote the metabolism and development of connective tissue and enhance blood flow, synthesis of collagen, wound repair, skin elasticity, and skin firmness.

Horsetail is high in vegetal silica and has been used since ancient Roman and Greek times. Organic silica promotes linking of collagen fibers and wound healing. Horsetail strengthens connective tissue and promotes the production of collagen and elastin. It stabilizes and strengthens tissue, improves circulation, and boosts regeneration of skin cells.

Licorice contains glycyrahizinic acid and flavonoids and is used as an anti-inflammatory and also for contact dermatitis. Licorice is used in contemporary DIY skin products to improve elasticity of the skin and to help in wound healing. It is also used as a skin lightener to even out skin tone and reduce hyperpigmentation.

....

Tip: There are a large variety of cosmeceuticals available for purchase. The variety of options may be overwhelming. To start, pick the skin condition that you want to treat, such as hyperpigmentation or fine lines. Purchase an ingredient that is reported to treat the condition and blend it with an OTC retail product or with a homemade cream. Use it consistently for about six weeks, the time that it takes for new cells to move to the surface of your skin. Take a before photo and take another after six weeks of treatment to monitor changes.

SKIN REJUVENATION

There are many DIY skin rejuvenation techniques and tools that can be used at home, enabling you to select the ones that best fit your skin care philosophy, budget, and routine.

DIY facial exercise, massage, and other treatments can make small improvements in the short term and more substantial improvements in the long term with consistent practice. With few exceptions, most DIY skin care rejuvenation tools or devices are not as powerful as the devices used by plastic surgeons, dermatologists, medical spas, or aestheticians. However, with consistent long-term use, DIY skin care treatments can be effective with noticeable results.

This section provides a brief summary of popular DIY skin care treatments for home use and does not discuss treatments used by professional dermatologists and medical spas.

Advantages of using DIY skin care treatments include:

*   convenience and flexible schedule
*   low costs
*   ability to combine techniques for personal needs

The treatments described below range from DIY skin care routines to devices that enhance the quality of your skin.

FACIAL EXPRESSIONS

You can change how you look and how you appear to the world by changing your facial expression and wearing a slight smile instead of a frown. Scientists used to think that your brain and happy thoughts make you smile. Studies have shown that the act of smiling can change your brain and make you healthier and happier. Develop a new and beneficial habit by slightly smiling with your face and eyes throughout each day for three weeks until it becomes a new normal for you. A smiling face looks more youthful than a frown!

Repetitive muscle contractions eventually damage muscle fibers and the overlying skin tissue resulting in deep lines. To minimize development of permanent wrinkles, practice maintaining a serene, slightly smiling, expression on your face to avoid making unconscious and consistent facial expressions that result in unwanted deep facial lines. For example, over time furrowing your eyebrows can lead to the development of lines, referred to as a "1" or "11" lines, in between your eyebrows. It is possible to change this habit by becoming conscious of your facial expressions and by relaxing your forehead muscles to keep them smooth.

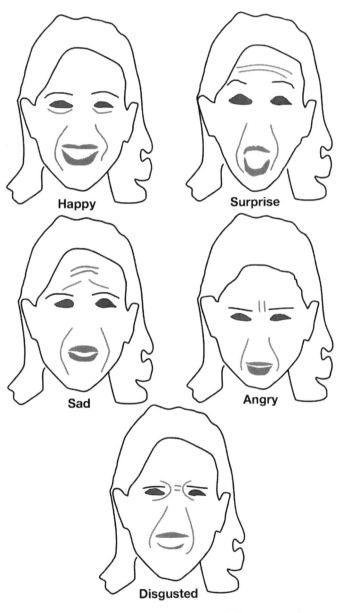

Happy

Surprise

Sad

Angry

Disgusted

Dynamic wrinkles during facial expressions

Tip: Notice your personal facial expressions and how they impact your muscles and skin. Try to maintain a serene expression with a slight smile at all times. Seriously. This technique has worked for me for years. That the practice has now become a habit makes me especially grateful. So smile. This will help to soften fine lines and wrinkles and increase the happy cells in your brain. It will look great on you and is so much better than accidently wearing a scowl or a frown.

FACIAL WRINKLE PADS

Facial wrinkle pads provide an effective, non-invasive treatment for wrinkles and can be used to retrain facial muscles. There are a variety of facial pads on the market that have a wide price range. Facial pads have a simple design and the various brands function in a similar manner: when applied they temporarily immobilize the muscle so that it cannot contract.

When you wear facial pads and learn what it feels like to relax the muscle in a smooth, rather than a contracted state, you can teach yourself to keep the muscle relaxed and smooth when you're not wearing a facial pad.

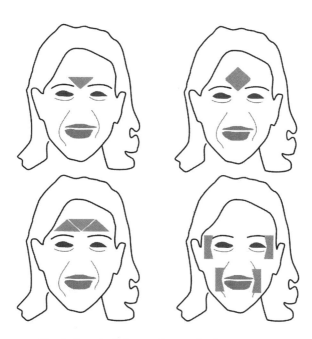

Facial wrinkle pads and placement

Facial pads are pre-cut pieces with adhesive on one side. To apply, use the fingers of one hand to spread the wrinkled skin and muscle beneath and position the facial pad on the area using the other hand. Wear the facial pad overnight or for at least three hours to allow the muscle to relax and smooth and to reduce the appearance of lines in the skin.

....

Tip: This is an easy way to diminish the appearance of facial lines and a good way to experience the feeling of the relaxed muscle when it is immobilized for hours. Initially, treated lines will be diminished when a facial pad is removed and with time, reappear. Consistent use of facial pads will result in progressive softening of facial lines.

MASSAGE

Massage has been used since ancient times for healing purposes. Facial massage is used to promote relaxation and restore energy by increasing circulation. Facial massage releases tension, minimizes the appearance of fine lines and wrinkles, promotes lymphatic flow, and increases skin radiance. Two types of facial massage are described below, friction massage and lymphatic massage.

Tip: Massage is an easy method to instantly brighten your complexion. Take five minutes to pinch, squeeze, pat, or twist your face and neck skin to get the circulation flowing for an immediate glow.

Friction Massage

Friction massage consists of vigorously rubbing the skin over a contracted muscle and is described by Sanford Bennett in the book *Exercising in Bed: The Simplest and Most Effective System of Exercise Ever Devised* published in 1907. Bennett was ill at the age of 50 when he developed an exercise program that restored his health and made him look younger at 72 than he had at 50. Bennett promoted facial exercise and friction massage, which uses the dry palms of the hands to vigorously massage the face and neck. Consistent vigorous massage over contracted muscles can be used to smooth forehead lines and a 1 or 11.

....

Tip: Friction massage is a regular part of my regimen. This massage stimulates the skin and will promote new skin cell growth. If you do this consistently, you will see a difference, especially in combination with facial exercise. These things take time. Practice the friction massage consistently for six weeks and monitor changes in your skin.

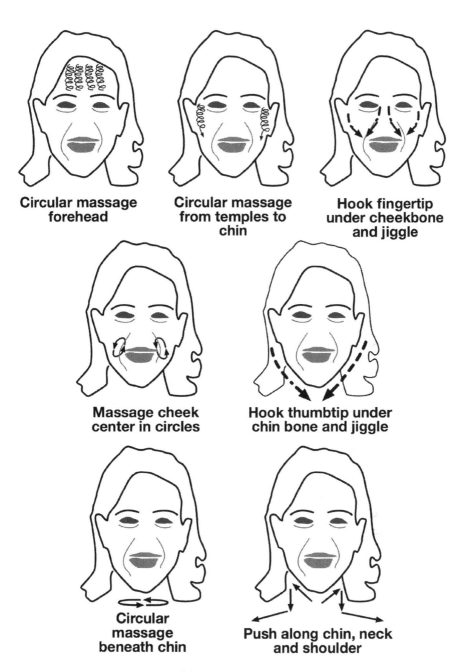

Circular massage forehead

Circular massage from temples to chin

Hook fingertip under cheekbone and jiggle

Massage cheek center in circles

Hook thumbtip under chin bone and jiggle

Circular massage beneath chin

Push along chin, neck and shoulder

Facial lymphatic massage

Lymphatic Massage

The lymph system removes and filters wastes from the bloodstream. The lymph does not have its own pump system and instead is stimulated by physical activity and massage. When the lymph is inactive, wastes accumulate. This can result in swelling or puffiness in the face. Facial massage stimulates the lymph system to flow properly, reducing puffiness. There are many written techniques and Internet video demonstrations for facial lymphatic massage. The lymphatic massage described by Karie Wagner at the All Natural Beauty website is fast, easy, and effective. After years of trying other methods, the lymphatic massage resulted in the elimination of my under-eye bags with consistent use. It only takes about five minutes to complete. The instructions suggest using the lymphatic massage every day for two weeks to jump-start the process and then cutting back to once a week for maintenance.

. . . .

Tip: As previously mentioned, lymphatic massage was the most effective treatment for eliminating my under eye puffiness, so simple, yet so effective. Based on how effective this method was at eliminating facial puffiness, use of this massage may also be effective for tightening skin loosened by congested facial lymph under the chin (sometimes referred to as "turkey neck").

FACIAL EXERCISE

Facial exercise provides a basic foundation for great skin. It works the muscles to fatigue, causing micro-injuries. As the micro-injuries heal, the muscles rebuild and become larger and stronger. Facial exercises may be done anywhere, they don't require special tools, and they can be completed in less than 30 minutes. Facial exercises can effectively maintain current muscle mass or build and strengthen shrunken or atrophied muscles, depending on the exercise methods used.

There are dozens of muscles in the face and neck. Because facial muscles connect to the skin, the health and condition of facial muscles have a direct impact on the appearance of the overlying skin. As facial muscles shrink and sag, the overlying skin sags too. When facial muscles are exercised and lifted, the skin is lifted.

When the skin is massaged and stimulated during facial exercise, skin cell turnover increases, as well as collagen and elastin production, resulting in soft, supple, and radiant skin. A contracted muscle increases circulation ten times. The increased circulation helps to remove wastes and bring in oxygen and nutrients, making the skin look terrific. The muscles on your face and neck function like the muscles of your body. For example, when you consistently use your muscles to run or lift weights, the muscle mass is maintained or increased. When you do not use your muscles, they lose mass and shrink. When you take a long break from exercising and then you begin again, your muscles will be weaker. If you continue to exercise, your muscles will get stronger.

The same is true for facial muscles. Eating and talking only exercise a portion of the facial muscles resulting in uneven muscle use and uneven muscle development, which promotes facial lines. If facial muscles are not exercised, they will sag, lose volume and strength, and the overlying skin will sag as well.

Deborah Crowley
FLEXEFFECT
flexeffect.com

Tom Hagerty
SHAPE YOUR FACE
shapeyourface.com

Charlotte Hamilton
FITFACE: THE NATURAL FACELIFT
fitfacetoning.com

Jeanette Johnson
FACE LIFTING EXERCISES
faceliftingexercises.com

Carole Maggio
FACERCISE
facercise.com

CYNTHIA ROWLAND
FACIAL MAGIC
cynthiarowland.com

Senta Maria Rungé
FACE LIFTING BY EXERCISE
faceliftingbyexercise.com

Fumiko Takatsu
FACE YOGA METHOD
faceyogamethod.com

Wendy Wilken
FACE ENGINEERING EXERCISES
face-engineering-exercises.org

Examples of facial exercise programs

My experience teaching facial exercise exposed me to a variety of students. Those who were in their twenties had strong facial muscles and were consistently sore the day after doing facial exercises. The older students whose facial muscles had atrophied might not be sore at all. When facial muscles atrophy or shrink, it takes time to rebuild them so it may take months before you can feel specific facial muscles contract during an exercise. Regardless, every time you do facial exercises your muscles and skin will benefit and if practiced consistently your facial muscles will build.

When men shave their face, they are unknowingly doing a form of facial exercise. They move their jaw from side to side, jut it out, and stretch the neck. These movements exercise the muscles and may be one reason why men seem to maintain good muscle tone as they age.

Facial exercises can be done using: low-level electrical stimulation devices, isometric exercises, and resistance training.

Tip: For me, facial exercise is one of the most effective ways to maintain muscle and bone strength and therefore, prevent skin sag. Try to make them part of your regular schedule. The increased circulation makes the skin look vibrant.

Isometric

Isometric exercises do not build new muscle mass but are terrific for maintaining current muscle strength and for increasing skin circulation. This type of exercise involves holding the facial muscles in a contracted state using a systematic set of expressions. There are dozens of isometric facial exercise programs available. Instructions on isometric facial exercises are easily available in books at libraries and bookstores and on the Internet.

Tip: Isometric exercises are a great way to start an exercise routine. They won't necessarily build new muscle, but they can maintain the muscle that you have. They can be done anywhere anytime because you don't need to use your hands or touch your face. You can do them at a stop light, watching TV, before falling asleep, sitting on the couch, when you wake up, or anywhere that you feel comfortable. They do involve making some funny faces.

Resistance

Resistance facial exercise involves contracting the facial muscles against resistance created using the hands and fingers to hold the muscles in place as they are contracted. Facial muscles are small and can be difficult to feel when you begin facial exercise, especially if your facial muscles are atrophied. Initially, you may not feel the effects of the resistance training, until you build your muscle strength. If you have good facial muscle strength, you will feel the muscle contract and your muscles may be sore after exercising. Resistance facial exercise significantly increases circulation, which is immediately evident by radiant skin.

If the facial muscles are atrophied it could take weeks, months, or even years to rebuild all of the facial muscles and to feel and see the full results of resistance facial exercise training. It is well worth it if you consider the alternative, which is continued facial muscle atrophy.

Tip: To see results, do resistant facial exercise for six months. Feel the changes in your muscles when you do facial massage. Take before and after photos. Watch for subtle changes in your forehead, eye area, cheeks, lips, chin, and neck. This process is not instantaneous it is cumulative and lasting.

DRY BRUSHING

Dry brushing is used to promote lymphatic circulation to remove toxins from the bloodstream, to increase skin circulation, and exfoliate dead skin cells. It consists of using a natural bristle body brush to vigorously brush the skin of the entire body, while dry, including the face and neck. Dry brushing begins at the body's extremities with brush strokes that move towards the heart. After dry brushing, an oil of your choice is massaged into the skin before rinsing with warm water.

Dry brushing increases skin stimulation, circulation, and removal of wastes. Removing dead skin cells promotes the production of new skin cells, which in turn causes the skin to become thicker. Be gentle when you begin; after your skin becomes accustomed to dry brushing, you'll be able to brush more vigorously for a terrific skin treatment experience! With continued use, vigorous skin treatments can make the skin stronger and more resilient.

Never dry brush over inflamed, tender, or irritated skin.

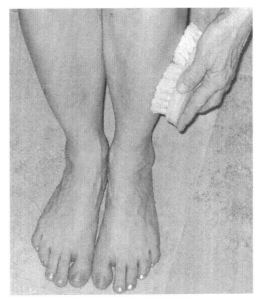

Dry brushing

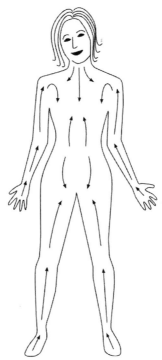

Lymphatic flow direction for dry brushing

Tip: Dry brushing helps to circulate wastes out of your bloodstream. It feels relaxing and revitalizing. Make a spa hour out of the occasion and dry brush, then use a sugar coconut oil scrub and spend time in a stream room for a healthy experience that feels indulgent.

CUPPING MASSAGE

Cupping massage is an ancient healing practice that uses suction on the skin to treat a variety of ailments. It is used to eliminate congestion, stagnation, blockages, toxins, and inflammation. Cupping improves circulation of blood and lymph and is used to detoxify the skin and the circulatory system.

In facial cupping massage, the skin is lubricated with oil and a suction cup is moved across the skin maintaining suction at all times. Contemporary cupping massage is typically done using glass cups and a rubber bulb that is squeezed to create suction or with cupped devices that use a battery operated pump to create a strong consistent suction.

Be gentle when using facial cupping massage; if the suction is too strong or a cup is held in one place for too long, this can result in a bruise on the skin. People who use facial cupping massage report their skin to be plumper, smoother, and firmer as a result.

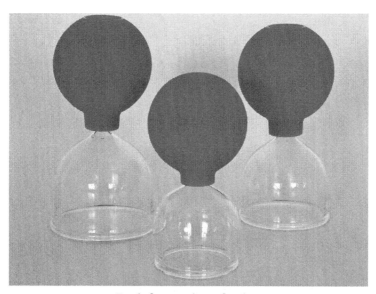

Facial cupping device

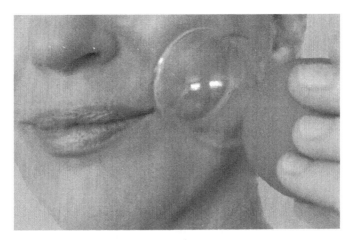

Facial cupping

Tip: This ancient healing practice has been integrated into skin care as another method to stimulate and improve the quality of the skin. It is important that you stimulate the skin. These different methods provide options to suit your lifestyle, time, and budget.

MICRODERMABRASION

Home microdermabrasion removes dead skin cells from the skin surface. Types of devices include vibrating devices that are used in conjunction with a granular exfoliating cream or vacuum devices that use diamond tips. The exfoliation gently removes dead skin cells from the skin surface. When microdermabrasion is used on a consistent basis it can promote a smooth, even appearance in skin tone. There are a variety of microdermabrasion devices in a range of prices that operate at varying strengths. Research the Internet for the type of device that would suit your needs for home use.

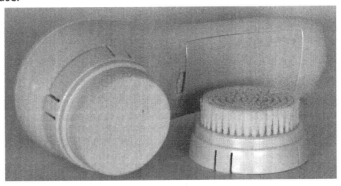

Microdermabrasion device

Microdermabrasion is used to treat hyperpigmentation and skin dullness. It also promotes product penetration. Microdermabrasion should not be used on keloidal scars or to remove skin growths.

....

Tip: Use microdermabrasion regularly. Even a microdermabrasion washcloth can be remarkably easy and effective. Use the washcloth after doing OCM or simply to freshen skin and enhance product penetration. A variety of microdermabrasion methods are readily available. Take the time to exfoliate your skin and afterwards, apply a cosmeceutical serum.

DERMAROLLING

Percutaneous collagen induction (PCI), dermarolling, and micro-needling all refer to a facial treatment developed in 1997 by Dr. Desmond Fernandes. PCI consists of a roller with small needles sticking out of it that is rolled across your skin. Different needle lengths are used for different purposes.

The needling device is rolled over the face and neck in a pattern that ensures sufficient penetration of the needles over the entire facial skin surface.

An important aspect of the PCI treatment is that the needles penetrate the skin intermittently, leaving the epidermis intact. This promotes faster healing times and allows the procedure to be repeated for optimal results. According to Fernandes, another advantage of PCI over other skin care treatments is that it does not cause hyperpigmentation and is safe to use on dark skin. With time, PCI skin rejuvenation noticeably improves the appearance of the skin as increased collagen and elastin production promote thicker skin. PCI needle lengths for home use range in size from 0.15 millimeter (mm) to 2.0 mm.

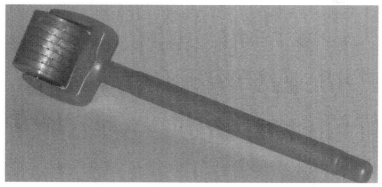

Dermaroller with short needles

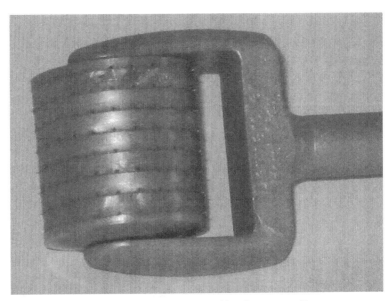

Close up of short needle dermaroller

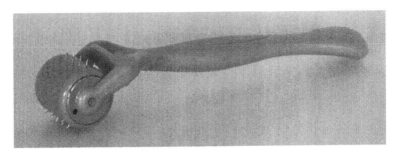

Long needle dermaroller

Shorter needles, from 0.15 to 0.5 mm, are used to enhance penetration of active ingredients. Short needles are primarily used to open shallow channels in the epidermis to dramatically increase the ability of active products to penetrate into the dermis and maximize the effectiveness of cosmeceutical ingredients. Short needles do not reach nerve endings and typically do not cause pain.

Short needle PCI treatments can be done every day depending on how sensitive your skin is and the type of active products that are applied. Due to the skin's increased absorption, it is important to select skin care products that are non-allergenic and contain non-irritating, high quality ingredients.

Longer needles, from 0.5 to 1.5 mm, penetrate the epidermis and the dermis to create intermittent micro injuries. These micro injuries initiate a cascade of biological healing processes that produce a connective tissue network that is comprised of collagen and elastin. Increased collagen and elastin production results in firmer and thicker skin. The channels close up a few hours after needling.

Needles longer than 1.5 mm are available, however they are typically used at home for body needling of stretch marks or in a dermatologist's office with anesthesia for deeper facial needling.

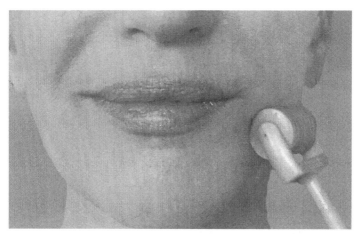

Facial dermaroller

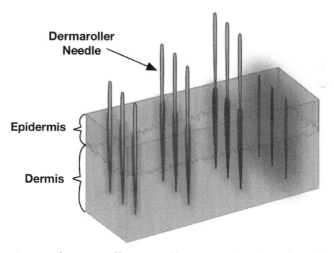

Long dermaroller needles penetrating the skin

To enhance deep PCI collagen production, pre-treat the skin with vitamins A and C for at least three weeks prior to the treatment and consistently after the treatment. After a deep PCI treatment, products penetrate the skin easily and less aggressive products should be used. It is best to use special formulations of fat-soluble vitamin A and C solutions after a PCI treatment because they are less irritating to the skin than the water-soluble vitamin C and Retin-A products.

When using longer needles to promote collagen production, multiple DIY PCI treatments provide the best results. Practitioners typically recommend three to six treatments a year when using rollers with needle lengths of 1.0 mm to 1.5 mm. There is controversy regarding the frequency of deep PCI treatments. Some experts recommend that deeper treatments be spaced out every two weeks and others suggest waiting a minimum of four to six weeks between each treatment.

Deep PCI rolls can be uncomfortable. The skin is typically numbed prior to a deep roll. After a deep PCI roll, monitor your skin's progress before deciding when to schedule your next deep roll. Allow time for the biologic healing cascade and collagen production process to proceed.

To numb the skin, ice or numbing cream may be used. If using ice, leave the ice in contact with the skin for five to seven minutes. Anything longer than 10 minutes can damage the skin. If a numbing cream is used, apply it thickly over the area to be rolled. Plastic is then placed over the cream to keep it moist during numbing. The numbing cream is wiped off prior to rolling.

EMLA numbing cream (lidocaine 2.5 percent and prilocaine 2.5 percent), is sometimes used before getting a tattoo or receiving a medical injection, and is often used for deep PCI rolls. A prescription is required to obtain EMLA. EMLA may be purchased from Internet pharmacies that will contact your physician for a prescription. Internet pharmacy transactions are professional and the EMLA price is competitive. If you buy EMLA online, compare prices or ask your physician for a prescription and buy it from a local pharmacy.

PCI provides a safe alternative to effectively treat hyperpigmentation, fine lines, wrinkles and scars and for smoothing the skin. Fernandes reports that six months after a deep PCI treatment, there is about a 400 percent increase in collagen and elastin in the skin.

Do not use PCI if you have skin conditions that require medical treatment; if you have active acne or other skin outbreaks; if you form keloid scars; are on blood thinning therapies; are receiving high levels of corticosteroids, chemotherapy or radiotherapy; or have uncontrolled diabetes mellitus.

Tip: This is my favorite device because it is so effective. Whether you use short needles to increase product penetration or long needles to stimulate collagen and elastin production, this is a winner. There are many striking before and after photos on the Internet illustrating the effectiveness of dermarolling. You can use this method yourself at home or, if you prefer, you may be able to find a clinic nearby to do it for you, at a price. Regardless, this is a great way to maintain thick skin. The difference is apparent two to three months after treatment.

Radiofrequency

Radiofrequency is used to tighten and lift sagging skin. It delivers electrical pulses and heat energy into the middle and lower levels of the skin and physically changes the skin's molecular structure. Following radiofrequency treatments, the wound healing process results in the growth of new collagen and skin tissue that slowly tightens over time.

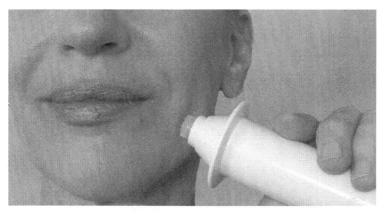

<u>**Radiofrequency device for home use**</u>

Radiofrequency is used as a non-surgical method to tighten the skin and also to destroy fat cells, which support and protect facial skin. Some folks have concern about the potential to lose supportive facial fat during a radiofrequency treatment. Radiofrequency devices are available for home use but people who have used the devices report mixed results. Testimonial before-and-after photos illustrate that radiofrequency treatments can result in skin-tightening. Results of radiofrequency have been unpredictable and can vary for different individuals.

Tip: The DermaWand is a low-amplitude, 168,000 microcurrent device that uses radiofrequency technology for home skin treatments. Used properly, it can effectively eliminate blemishes, reduce puffy eyes, and oxygenate your skin. Have fun exploring while you identify your optimum personal skin care treatments.

LIGHT EMITTING DIODES

Light consists of photon movement that produces electromagnetic (EM) waves. The spectrum of EM waves includes radio waves, infrared radiation, visible light, ultraviolet rays, x-rays, gamma rays, and cosmic radiation.

Light emitting diodes (LED) were developed by NASA to grow plants in space. Subsequent testing showed that use of LED treatments resulted in a 40 percent improvement in healing time for injuries by increasing cell growth 150 to 200 percent in treated areas. Further analyses showed that light travels 23 centimeters into skin and muscle at wavelengths of 630 to 800 nanometers (nm). Astronauts who are subjected to prolonged weightlessness experience a decline in bone and muscle mass. NASA investigations showed that use of LEDs stimulated wound healing and tissue regeneration and quintupled the growth of fibroblasts and muscle cells in tissue culture. Super LEDs are becoming more popular because they are brighter.

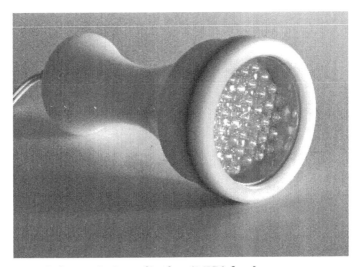

Light emitting diodes (LED) for home use

Different color LEDs are used for different skin treatments. For example, blue (407 to 420 nm) and red (633 to 660 nm) lights are used to treat acne, and red and yellow (588 nm) are used as anti-aging treatments to increase collagen production. Red and near infrared light within 600 to 1,000 nm wavelengths promote healing of the skin by promoting fibroblast proliferation, synthesis of collagen types I and II, and accelerated tissue repair. It appears that light wave doses ranging from 1.0 to 6.0 Joule per square centimeter promote faster healing. Use this information when purchasing an LED for home use to ensure that you get a device that operates in the range necessary to treat your skin care concerns.

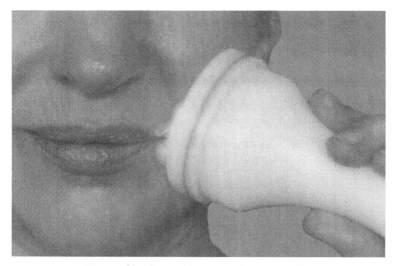

<u>Use of light emitting diode (LED)</u>

Studies show that LED treatments using a combination of 633 nm and 830 nm (red and infrared) resulted in "a statistically significant improvement in wrinkles" over a 12-week period of time. Test subjects reported softer, smoother, and firmer skin and analyses showed that collagen fibers were thicker after treatment. Studies also show that age spots may be lightened using LED photo rejuvenation.

Use of LED devices in home skin care can result in the development of new collagen, promote skin rejuvenation, and have anti-aging effects. Light is absorbed and stored as energy, which is later used in the biological processes required to repair tissue.

....

Tip: NASA studies showed the healing benefits associated with the use of LEDs. To increase collagen and elastin, use an LED with infrared and red lights to augment your facials. You may like it so much that you will follow the author's lead and install LED lights in your bathroom to create an LED treatment room.

ELECTRICAL MUSCLE STIMULATION

Electrical muscle stimulation (EMS) uses low voltage electrical currents to contract muscles, which increases circulation and prevents muscle atrophy by exercising, building, and strengthening the muscles. An EMS may be used as a facial exercise routine. EMS devices include galvanic and microcurrent.

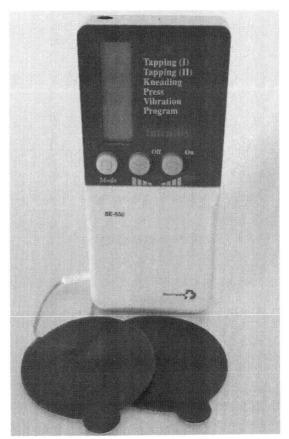

Electrical muscle stimulation device

Tip: This is a good method to use to simulate your facial muscles. Use of this device introduced me to facial exercises which led me to muscle strength training.

Galvanic

Galvanic devices apply a constant high voltage, low amperage, unidirectional microcurrent to the skin that stimulates deep tissue circulation, promotes wound healing, and pore cleansing. Galvanic microcurrent may be operated using either negative or positive charges. The negative charge is used to clean skin via desencrustation. The positive charge is used to deliver active ingredients into the skin via iontophoresis.

Desencrustation is used to clean the skin by liquefying sebum (skin oil), make-up residues, and wastes that are present in hair follicles and pores. The process softens the skin and increases circulation in the treatment area.

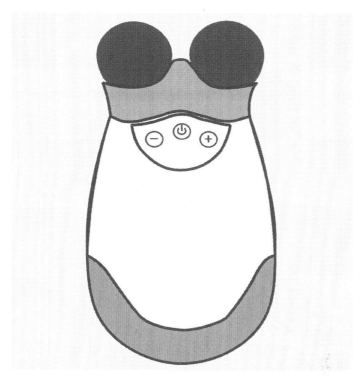

Galvanic microcurrent device

Iontophoresis enhances product penetration by decreasing the pH and increasing the permeability of the skin. It increases penetration of water-soluble active serums, liquids, and gels into the skin for enhanced rejuvenation. Iontophoresis has been used clinically for decades to deliver medication into the body. Iontophoresis reduces inflammation and can reduce swelling when the skin is irritated from the use of other facial treatments, to help the skin look better sooner.

....

Tip: Add a galvanic device to your skin care tool collection and be prepared to pull wastes out, push nutrient serums in, and enjoy invigorated skin. To liquefy skin oils that clog pores, use the negative electrode with a blend of distilled water and 10 percent baking soda.

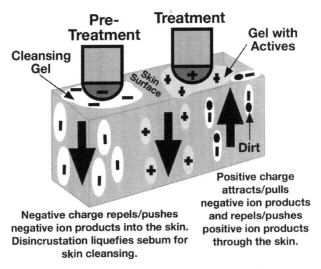

Negative charge repels/pushes negative ion products into the skin. Disincrustation liquefies sebum for skin cleansing.

Positive charge attracts/pulls negative ion products and repels/pushes positive ion products through the skin.

Galvanic microcurrent penetration

Microcurrent

Microcurrent uses small electric currents that are measured in millionths of an ampere, or microamperes (µA). Microcurrent is referred to as biostimulation or bioelectricity because it mimics cellular level electrical processes that occur during energy synthesis of adenosine triphosphate (ATP) and proteins. Currents below 500 µA increase ATP, which maintains the health of the cell membrane, waste management, and promotes collagen synthesis. Bioelectricity is used to alter cellular activity to enhance healing of the skin by speeding up the rate of cellular biological processes.

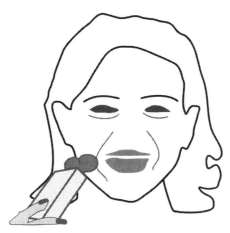

Use of microcurrent device

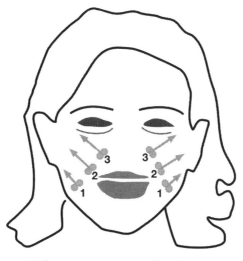

Microcurrent application

. . . .

Tip: Microcurrent could be your favorite tool; with regular use the impulses can tone the face and neck, stimulate lymph flow, increase circulation and product penetration, exfoliate the skin, and minimize sun damage. Results may vary.

ULTRASOUND

Ultrasound, also known as sonophoresis or phonophoresis, utilizes high frequency sound waves, referred to as ultrasonic waves, to penetrate water-soluble active gels and serums into the skin for enhanced facial rejuvenation. Ultrasound decreases skin pH thereby increasing skin permeability and product penetration.

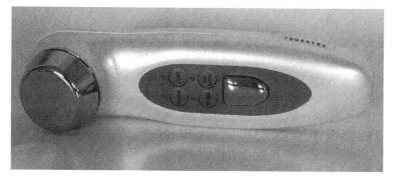

Ultrasound device

Studies show that low frequency ultrasound enhances delivery of active ingredients into the skin. The process is not thoroughly understood, but it is believed that the ultrasonic waves produce thermal, mechanical, and chemical changes. For example, ultrasound waves change the fats or lipids in the stratum corneum, which may enhance product penetration.

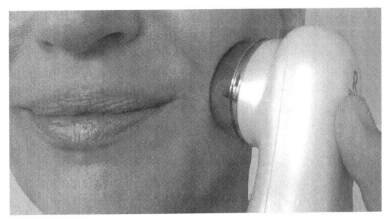

Use of ultrasound device

Thermal effects create friction and increase local heat promoting metabolism of biocellular components used in the production of collagen, elastin, and connective tissue. The increased temperature stimulates blood flow, which increases delivery of oxygen and nutrients used for healing and increases lymph flow to aid in the removal of toxins and waste products. The mechanical effects of ultrasound include tissue massage, increased tone and elasticity of the skin, and softening of scars.

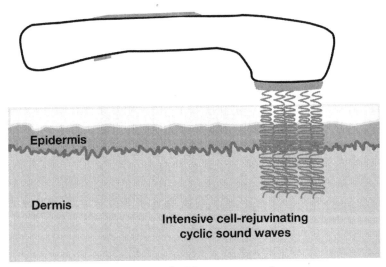

Ultrasound skin penetration

Low-frequency sonophoresis can be used to enhance penetration of matrixyl and other peptides. Research has found that the use of ultrasound can stimulate fibroblasts, increase local circulation, and stimulate wound repair.

Ultrasound devices come in different strengths. The lower the ultrasound frequency, the deeper the penetration. A three-megahertz (MHz) device provides shallow penetration of ultrasound waves, while one MHz and two MHz ultrasound frequencies penetrate deeper.

All three frequencies may be used for body and facial skin treatments. The one MHz sound waves target the middle layer of the skin dermis where collagen, elastin, and DNA are manufactured. The sound waves increase the metabolism of collagen and elastin production, creating healthier, thicker, firmer, and more youthful skin. A one MHz device with variable settings allows for superficial and deep penetration of active ingredients and enhanced rejuvenation of the skin for the face and body.

Ultrasound therapy has a long history of safe, successful use for physical therapy and wound healing. Currently, the level of ultrasound frequency used in DIY skin care is controversial. Some proponents say that three MHz devices are best suited for facial skin care, while other proponents say that one MHz devices are best suited for facial skin. Both types of devices are available for purchase and are being used for DIY facial skin care.

....

Tip: The ultrasound devices that are available for home use are not as powerful as those in a physician's office, but they do deliver an effective treatment. Ultrasound can enhance delivery of nutraceutical products into the skin. Trim the scratchy edges of an aloe vera leaf, slice the leaf down the middle, apply the gel to your face and neck then follow with ultrasound. This technique enhances collagen production and results in glowing skin.

LASER

DIY laser devices for skin rejuvenation are an emerging market. Lasers produce a beam of concentrated light with high energies. These energies promote the production of cell biology energy and growth factors that result in the generation of new tissue. There are several DIY laser devices used for skin rejuvenation.

Ablative laser technology removes the entire epidermis, requires longer healing times, and results in dramatic skin improvement. Ablative laser technology is not available for home use.

In recent years, nonablative laser technology was developed to treat small, intermittent portions of the epidermis while leaving some portions of the epidermis undamaged to support faster healing times and to protect against infection. Nonablative laser treatments target deep skin layers and promote skin rejuvenation.

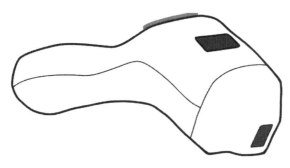

Laser device for home use

In cosmetic dermatology, nonablative fractional lasers are used in the range of 1064, 1320, 1450, and 1540 nm to improve uneven skin texture and to reduce the appearance of fine wrinkles and scarring.

In recent years, nonablative low-level laser devices have become available for home use. Some of these devices have received FDA approval, but do not have a long history of use and results. At this time, it is best to research Internet skin care boards to read reviews by skin care enthusiasts who have used particular devices before purchasing your own device.

One such device is targeted to treat eye wrinkles and operates at approximately 1410 nm, pulses for 10 milliseconds, and has a maximum energy output of 15 millijoules. Results based on use of this device are mixed. Similar to other skin rejuvenation treatments, laser results are not immediate. It takes months to observe the effects of these treatments on collagen and elastin production.

If you easily develop hyperpigmentation, precautions should be taken before using a laser device. Pretreat the skin for four weeks by applying actives that suppress melanin production. After nonablative laser treatments, the skin may be red and swollen and may have pinpoint bleeding depending on the intensity of the treatment.

....

Tip: Research skin care message boards to read the most recent opinions regarding use of home laser devices. If you decide to try one, ask if you should pretreat for hyperpigmentation before use.

DEBORAH'S LIFESTYLE

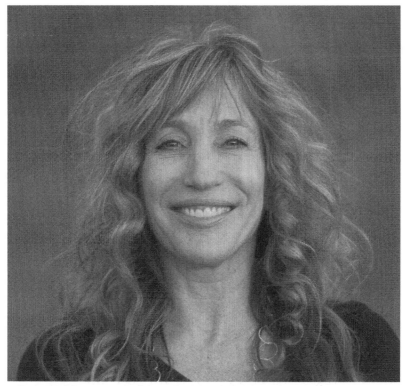

Chris McPherson Photography http://chrismcpherson.com

The lifestyle that I enjoy promotes good health, which is beautiful. Lifestyle practices can also be used to improve the quality of your skin.

My lifestyle choices are based on my primary goal to feel my best each day. Practices that I integrate into my life include:

- high quality food
- consistent exercise
- stretching for flexibility
- strength and balance
- meditation
- a positive attitude
- hard work
- good rest
- friends and family
- sufficient sleep

The more balanced I am in these areas, the better my mood and energy levels. These are the things that I have in my control that I can use to achieve a high quality of life, feel my best, and be ready for new experiences. There are many side benefits to a healthy lifestyle including physical strength, fitness endurance, increased brainpower, and a great foundation for healthy skin!

To me, beautiful skin has a velvety soft appearance. I believe that a healthy lifestyle can help nurture and maintain velvety skin.

I began learning about nutrition in the late 1970s and continue to learn and modify my eating habits today. The foundation of my diet is high quality, whole, unprocessed, organic food. I developed my healthy eating habits based on research, instinct, and how I feel after eating.

Over time, my eating and cooking patterns evolved. I integrate healthy ingredients into my favorite recipes by replacing refined grains with whole unprocessed grains, reducing the sugar and salt content, and using healthy fats. For example, when modifying a baking recipe, I replace most or all of the white flour with whole wheat flour, brown rice flour or coconut flour. These are only a few suggestions; there are many other whole grains and flours that may be substituted for white flour.

In 1990 while in my early 30s, I began buying organic food grown without synthetic pesticides and fertilizers to minimize my daughter and my ingestion of chemicals and to support sustainable agricultural technologies to protect the environment.

It was not an easy decision to buy organic because of the high cost, however I made a choice to spend my money on what I considered to be the best food available. I chose not to buy extra material goods so that I could purchase local and organic foods. My biggest investment in my daughter's, my own, and the earth's health has been buying whole organic foods. Along these lines, I also avoid exposing myself to chemicals in other areas of my life whenever I can. I am grateful to be able to vote with my dollar and buy food that is grown using sustainable practices and without chemicals.

In 1991, I chose to boycott the meat industry over its treatment of animals and became a vegetarian. Seven years later, I craved salmon for a year and I began eating fish. I continue to eat fish periodically—less than five percent of the time—and I try to select sustainably harvested fish whenever possible. I have not eaten meat for 23 years and have never craved it. More recently, I increased the amount of vegan (no animal products) and raw (uncooked or cooked below 104 degrees Fahrenheit) options in my diet. I also experimented with reducing or excluding grains from my diet and increasing my protein consumption.

Also, in the early 1990s, I stopped eating fat as was the trend and for a few years I ate my toast dry. Now I eat loads of good fats and my health and skin are better because of it. My current favorite fat is unrefined, raw, organic coconut oil. It smells divine and tastes great by the spoonful, so you can imagine how a cookie baked with coconut oil tastes—super yummy!

I drank soda as a child but stopped when I was 18 and for decades, I only drank water and a cup or two of coffee daily. Around 2007, I tried Kombucha and instinctively knew it was good for me and I continue to drink it today. I primarily drink water, one or two strong cups of coffee in the morning, two to four cups of green tea a day, and a periodic cup of Kombucha. In 2009, I began juicing vegetables one week a month using greens, celery, carrots, apples, ginger, garlic and parsley. I began juicing daily in 2013 and continue to drink about 20 ounces of green juice a day. I enjoy a glass of champagne or sparkling wine on occasion; however I may go months without an alcoholic drink.

I do not drink fruit juice and I did not feed my daughter fruit juice because it contains high concentrations of fruit sugars that can rapidly raise glucose levels. It is best to eat the whole fruit rather than drink fruit juice because the fruit fiber slows down digestion of the fruit sugars.

I have taken nutraceuticals for about 20 years. I take anti-oxidants and anti-inflammatory supplements to fight free radicals and to reduce inflammation. I regularly take vitamin C, beta-carotene (converts to vitamin A), vitamin E (a blend of tocotrienols and tocopherols), and zinc. I also take vitamin B for stress, fish oil (tested for mercury) for essential fatty acids, and a high quality multi-vitamin.

I take additional supplements based on how I feel, my health needs, and my finances. For example, a few years ago I added calcium, magnesium, and vitamin D supplementation for general health. I sometimes take additional vitamins for skin care such as coenzyme Q-10, alpha lipoic acid, and DMAE. I recently began taking vitamin K supplements.

I currently take a suite of vitamins in the morning and a suite in the evening. To make it easier to take them every day and for when I travel, I sort and package my daily vitamins every two weeks. I take periodic breaks from consuming vitamins, such as one or two days off a week or one week off a month. I educate myself before choosing to integrate a nutraceutical into my routine.

In my teens and young adulthood, I was naturally active playing racquetball, hiking, and taking dance classes. When I became pregnant with my daughter at 29, I was compelled to be physically active every day. During my pregnancy, I began walking daily until the summer heat of Phoenix, Arizona, became too hot. I switched to riding a bicycle until my belly was too big to peddle comfortably. I transitioned to swimming one mile three times a week, which I did throughout my pregnancy until the day I delivered. Two weeks after my daughter's birth in 1988, I began swimming and walking again and have maintained a consistent exercise program since. I speed walk four miles a day or do an equivalent one-hour of cardio exercise six days a week. I push myself harder a few times a week to further boost my heart rate. I lift heavy things while gardening or working on the house. I cross-train by doing a variety of cardio exercises including hiking and biking. In the mid-1990's, I began practicing yoga and I still maintain a weekly yoga routine. Yoga increases flexibility, strength, relaxation, balance, and circulation. Exercise makes me feel great and that is why I do it. The additional benefits I get from consistent exercise are a bonus.

I practice and promote family exercise. I enjoy time together with family and friends while doing something fun and active. I pushed my daughter in a stroller and later in a jogger until she was seven and told me that she was embarrassed to ride in the jogger. Soon after that, she began riding her bike while I speed-walked. A few years later, my daughter began walking with me. During our daily exercise time together, she talked about her day and her life without the distraction of a radio, telephone, television, or computer. It was a great way to spend an hour with her. Now that she has graduated from college, we still exercise together whenever possible and she consistently exercises on her own. I am grateful that we can share exercise and that she has healthy habits to help her in life.

Although I work hard at my career and on personal projects I incorporate rest and good sleep habits into my lifestyle. I have quiet time, a consistent bedtime, and blackout curtains. I am flexible, as life requires, but I know that sleep is good for my health. If I struggle with my sleep, I try to envision images of peaceful places and I do not focus on my thoughts. If I can't sleep, I may take N-acetyl-5-methoxytryptamine (melatonin) or 5-hydroxytryptophan (5-HTP) tablets.

Melatonin is a hormone found naturally in the body and a synthetic supplement. Melatonin is most commonly available in pill form and may be effective in reducing the time that it takes to fall asleep. 5-HTP is involved in the biosynthesis of serotonin, which promotes relaxation and a feeling of well-being. I try to regularly get seven to eight hours of good sleep, which makes me feel fantastic and makes my skin look its best.

A positive mental attitude makes a beneficial difference in our lives. It is important to recognize one's own personal value especially when faced with those who give you undue criticism, a lack of respect, or are indifferent.

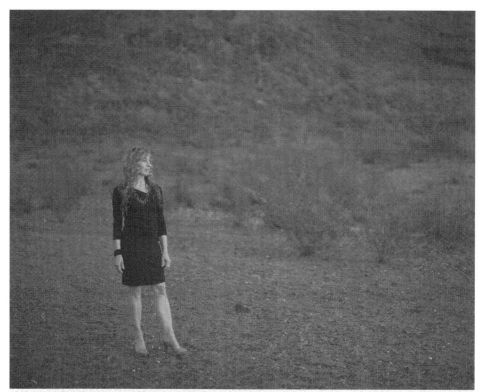

Chris McPherson Photography http://chrismcpherson.com

For many years I had poor self-confidence. Then I read that one must have compassion, patience, and tolerance for oneself before one can have these values towards others. That day, I decided to treat myself with more kindness and to stop being so judgmental towards myself. I am grateful that I have the opportunity to try and grow as a person throughout my life.

I avoid people who are demeaning and disrespectful. I love to be around positive people who are supportive and I try to be supportive as well.

It's imperative to have a positive outlook for optimum health.

DEBORAH'S SKIN CARE GOALS AND ROUTINE

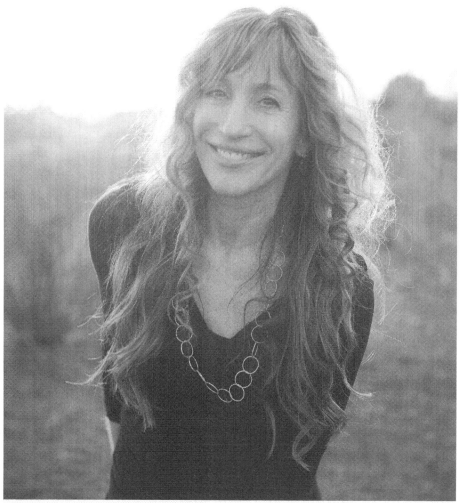

Chris McPherson Photography http://chrismcpherson.com

The skin care products and routines that I use are based on my skin care needs, my budget, and the amount of time that I have. I provide my personal routine as an example of a DIY cosmetic dermatology practice. My routine may not work for you. Learn about different DIY skin care practices to develop your personalized DIY skin care program.

I have worked as a geologist and hydrogeologist throughout my career. I did extensive fieldwork in southern Arizona during my early 20s. Some days, I was outside from dawn to dusk. I began covering my skin using sunscreen, hats, scarves, gloves, long sleeved shirts, long pants, and umbrellas. I also began using these sun protection practices in my personal life. I use an umbrella, rain or shine, for walking through parking lots, across campuses, or through downtown city centers. I use full coverage bathing suits and swim gloves when snorkeling. I keep a pair of gloves and a scarf in my car and wear them while driving. It may not be a sexy look, but my skin is in good shape because of it!

I live in one of the sunniest places on earth, southern Arizona, and I apply sunscreen to my face, neck, chest, and hands daily, year round, rain or shine. I primarily use a physical sunblock that contains zinc oxide and titanium dioxide. Chemical sunscreens irritate my skin, particularly when my skin is sensitive from DIY treatments. For many years, I did not use sunscreen on my chest and I developed hyperpigmentation. I began to use sunscreen and scarves to protect my chest from sun exposure. After three years, the hyperpigmentation on my chest began to fade. With time, I was able to reverse the sun damage on my chest. I was rewarded for my sun protection efforts when a dermatologist told me, "Your skin is amazing…you take phenomenal care of it." Despite my sun avoidance, my vitamin D level is at the top of the desired range.

I began giving myself facials in my 20s. I made my facial masks using ingredients that were readily available to me from my kitchen including yogurt, honey, and avocado. In my 30s, I made masks using ingredients purchased from health food stores, including brewer's yeast, vitamin E, and clay. In about 2001, in my 40s, my DIY skin care system became more sophisticated when I found skin care recipes on the Internet and began blending my own high concentration active skin care products. I started adding vitamins and herbal supplements to store bought creams. In 2002, I began making a vitamin C serum. My recipe has evolved over time and I still use the serum daily. In about 2006, I found DIY skin care message boards on the Internet as well as online merchants who sell cosmeceutical ingredients. I began blending these active ingredients into serums, lotions, and creams.

I began using devices for skin care in 2000 when I was 41. I had seen a TV infomercial for an electrical device that stimulated facial muscles. I was not a TV shopper but I was intrigued. I did not buy the device, which I later regretted because my instinct told me that exercising my facial muscles was a good idea. Later I stumbled across an electrical stimulation device at a home and garden show and bought it. I used the device consistently for a few months and after I saw positive results, I became devoted to facial exercise.

With time, I found the electrical muscle stimulation device time-consuming and awkward to use and I looked for another way. I found facial exercise books at used bookstores and this led me to begin practicing isometric exercises. With time, I wanted a more rigorous workout. I began facial resistance training in 2002 and I continue the exercises today. I was able to feel and see my facial muscles get stronger.

In about 2006, I began purchasing additional devices for DIY skin care treatments. I vary my recipes and routine based on information that I find on the Internet, my current skin care interests, and the active ingredients and devices that I have available to me.

I know that I am not going to eliminate the wrinkles around my eyes or crow's feet. I don't mind my crinkly eyes, but if I can maintain or improve the quality of my face and neck muscles and skin, I will. I accept the aging process but I would like to age gracefully.

My current daily skin care routine includes:

MORNINGS

- rinse face and neck with cool water
- use OCM only if my skin is peeling from a treatment
- apply DIY glucosamine/niacinamide serum, let dry or wait five minutes
- apply DIY water soluble vitamin C serum, let dry or wait five minutes
- apply DIY collagen building and skin firming cream
- apply sunscreen rain or shine, whether I am inside or outside, year round
- apply mineral makeup

EVENINGS

- use OCM every night or two to three nights a week
- use microfiber cloth on face and neck daily
- use 0.1 percent Retin-A two to three nights a week
- use oil soluble vitamin C and retinol two to three times a week
- use glycolic acid lotion once or twice a week

SKIN TREATMENTS THAT I ROUTINELY USE INCLUDE

- resistance facial exercises one to five times per week
- lymphatic massage, once weekly in the evening during the OCM
- friction massage, once weekly
- chemical and physical exfoliation, one to two times per week

- percutaneous collagen induction therapy (PCIT) or dermarolling using a short needle dermaroller to enhance product penetration, intermittently
- four to six annual PCIT treatments using a long needle dermaroller to increase collagen
- galvanic (iontophoresis)/ultrasound (sonophoresis or phonophoresis), during facials or after dermarolling
- periodic LED treatments
- periodic dermawand treatments

MY LIFESTYLE INCLUDES

- fresh whole foods from 1979
- an hour of hard cardio, six days a week from 1989
- cross-training from 1989
- organic foods from 1991
- dry or steam sauna once a week for minimum of 30 minutes from 1991
- a combination of vegetarian, vegan, and raw from 1992
- yoga from 1995
- pescatarian from 1999
- scheduling rest into my week whenever possible

During my first five years of facial exercise, I practiced resistance facial training six days a week. After achieving the results that I wanted, I reduced my workouts to about three times a week. There are no special tools required to practice facial resistance exercises. You only need your hands and a little bit of time. Facial exercises can be done anywhere. With age, facial muscles atrophy but can be strengthened with exercise to prevent muscle sagging. The benefits of facial exercise become more noticeable with time.

With resistance training, I am able to build and maintain muscle mass. When I began facial exercise, my muscles were weak and I could hardly feel them contract during exercise. With time, my facial muscles developed strength and now I can feel the muscles contract during my workout. I am devoted to practicing resistance facial exercise throughout my life. I exercise my body regularly and it makes sense to exercise my face as well.

I have a habit of needlessly furrowing my eyebrows. I began using facial pads around 2002 on the 1-line that I have in between my eyebrows. Regular use of facial pads has proven to be effective in minimizing furrow lines.

I use the dry brush method on my face, neck, and body. At first, it was intimidating to dry brush my face, but as my skin became stronger I became more confident.

Now I vigorously dry brush my face to strengthen my skin, make it more resilient, and increase circulation. For a special treat, I dry brush my face and body, apply a raw organic coconut oil sugar scrub, and lay on a towel in a sauna, going in and out over a period of about an hour. I then rinse, dry, and relax!

I tried the cupping massage a couple of times, but I have not integrated it into my daily skin care routine. I purchased glass cups with rubber suction bulbs on eBay. I found using the cups to be awkward but could see how it would become easier with practice. I choose to spend my time doing facial exercises instead of cupping because it has the added benefit of working the muscle.

I am in my seventh year of facial dermarolling treatments. I massaged my face and neck for seven years before beginning dermarolling and that helped me to know what my skin felt like pre-dermarolling. Six months after doing my first set of six dermarolling sessions in 2008, I could see the difference in my skin texture and I could feel that my skin had become thicker.

I regularly make the OCM cleanser, the glucosamine/niacinimide serum, a water-based vitamin C serum, an oil-based vitamin C and vitamin A serum, and a collagen building lotion. It takes me about two to four hours a month to make the DIY products I use, which maintain an even skin tone while nourishing my skin. My serums are high quality products that make a visible difference in my skin quality.

Periodically, I buy and use an expensive, high quality skin care product. I have found that products purchased OTC at retail outlets are rarely better and they are often inferior to the DIY products I make. With one exception, my favorite retail skin care products are made by Environ® developed by Dr. Desmond Fernandes who has made dramatic advances in cosmetic dermatology. He has dozens of before and after photos to illustrate his success.

I use a red and infrared LED device after I complete a deep dermarolling session. I was advised by an esthetician to use the LED after dermarolling because the procedure opens channels in the skin enabling better penetration of the LED lights. I believe that this device augments my skin care program, but I cannot distinguish the benefits of this device from other devices. Nor have I established a consistent treatment routine with this device to experience the optimum results.

I currently use ultrasound to push vitamin C serum and fresh aloe vera gel into my face and neck skin. I have not used my galvanic device yet.

Enhancing your skin care routine can be time consuming but a skin care program can be developed that suits your lifestyle. Choose a treatment that you can easily integrate into your routine and try it for a while. I consider the time that I spend on my facial program as spa time, which I use for relaxation and rejuvenation. Doing a facial is also a meditative practice for me.

Over time, I have developed a skin care routine that fits my schedule and is realistic for me to achieve. I am flexible and modify my routine to fit my lifestyle as required when my schedule changes. In the past, I did not have the money or time to visit the dermatologist, medical spa, or esthetician regularly. DIY cosmetic dermatology has enabled me to develop and use a high quality skin care routine. I receive compliments from men and women alike on the quality of my skin and I am grateful that there are high quality skin care options available for those on a budget.

I hope that the information in this book helps you develop a skin care routine that fits your lifestyle and results in radiant skin.

REFERENCES

Aesthetic Plastic Surgery, May-June 2000, pages 227-234; *Phytomedicine*, May 2001, pages 230-235; and *Contact dermatitis*, October 1993, pages 175-179.

Alam, M., & Dover, J.S., 2003. *Nonablative Laser and Light Therapy: An approach to patient and device selection*. http://www.skintherapyletter.com/2003/8.4/2.html, Volume 8 - 2003 TOC, accessed February 21, 2011.

Alcamo, I. E., 1997. *Anatomy coloring workbook*. Random House, Inc., New York, 1997. Pgs 204 to 206.

American Journal of Clinical Dermatology, March-April 2000, pages 81-88.

Aust MC, Reimers K, Repenning C, Stahl F, Jahn S, Guggenheim M, Schwaiger N, Gohritz A, Vogt PM., 2008. *Percutaneous collagen induction: minimally invasive skin rejuvenation without risk of hyperpigmentation-fact or fiction?* Plast Reconstr Surg. 2008 Nov;122(5):1553-63. Klinik für Plastische, Hand- und Wiederherstellungschirurgie, Medizinische Hochschule Hannover, Hannover, Germany. aust_matthias@gmx.de.

Banga, A.K., 1998. *Electrically assisted transdermal and topical drug delivery: metabolism and molecular physiology of saccharomyces*. Pgs: 185, Publisher: CRC Press, 06/1998.

Baumann, L., 2013. http://health.yahoo.net/experts/skintype/effects-stress-your-skin, accessed October 14, 2013.

Beanes, S.R., Dang, C., Soo, C., & Ting, K., 2003. *Skin repair and scar formation: the central role of TGF-[beta]*. Expert Reviews in Molecular Medicine/Volume 5/2003, pp 1-22, Copyright © Cambridge University Press 2003, DOI: http://dx.doi.org/10.1017/S1462399403005817, Published online: 13 February 2004, accessed March 7, 2011.

Bennett, S., 1907. *Exercising in bed the simplest and most effective system of exercise ever devised*. The Edward Hilton Co. Publishers.

Bissett, D. L., 2006. *Glucosamine: an ingredient with skin and other benefits*. J Cosmet Dermatol. 2006 Dec;5 (4):309-15.

Bogle, M. A. 2007, *Minimally invasive techniques for improving the appearance of the aging face*. Expert Review of Dermatology 2.4 (August 2007): p427(9). (7892 words).

Bradley, P.R. (ed.). 1992. *British herbal compendium*, Vol. 1. Bournemouth: British Herbal Medicine Association.

Brannon, Healther, 2007. *What causes wrinkles, normal skin & chronological aging*. About.com Guide, Updated January 14, 2007. http://dermatology.about.com/cs/

beauty/a/wrinklecause.htm, accessed April 9, 2011.

Braukus, M., Berg, J., 2003. *NASA light-emitting diode technology brings relief in clinical trials*. RELEASE : 03-366. November 13, 2003. http//www.msfc.nasa.gov/news.

Castor Oil Uses, 2011. *Castor oil uses, a comprehensive castor oil resource.* http://www.castoroilhome.com/castor-oil-benefits-need-to-know, accessed on July 14, 2011.

Chukuka S. Enwemeka, PT, PhD, FACSM, *Therapeutic light,* January/February 2004, http://www.rehabpub.com/features/1022004/2.asp, accessed March 7, 2011.

Copyright Thinkwell, All Rights Reserved, 2013. *Layers of the skin.* September 9, 2013.

Crowley, D., 2010. *FlexEffect facialbuilding.* FlexEffect Publishing, Eureka, CA. 2010.

D'Amelio, Frank S. Sr., *Botanicals, a phytocosmetic desk reference*, CRC Press, 1999.

Daily Green, 2011. *Dirty dozen foods.* http://www.thedailygreen.com/healthy-eating/eat-safe/dirty-dozen-foods#fblndex1, accessed September 5, 2011.

Daniels, R., 2004. *Strategies for skin penetration enhancement.* Skin Care Forum, Issue 37 — August 2004) scf-online.com | Issue 37 | Rolf Daniels_ Strategies for Skin Penetration Enhancement.pdf.

Dermatology Blog, 2008. *Do peptides in skin care products work.* http://thedermblog.com/2008/06/23/do-peptides-in-skin-care-products-work/, accessed June 26, 2011.

Environmental Working Group, EWG, 2011. http://www.ewg.org/, accessed September 5, 2011.

Essential Day Spa, 2011. *Essential Day Spa Forum.* http://www.essentialdayspa.com/forum/, accessed December 11, 2011.

Essential Day Spa, 2015. *Dr. Kassy's face firming and eye cream.* Essential Day Spa: Skincare Tools & Do-It-Yourself Skincare: Sticky: DIY Skin Care—Recipe Index, Dermarolling, Facial Exercise, thread: http://www.essentialdayspa.com/forum/viewthread.php?p=417200, accessed March 23, 2015.

Essential Day Spa, 2015. *Keliu's glucosamine & niacinamide serum, version A (2/29/09).* Essential Day Spa: Skincare Tools & Do-It-Yourself Skincare: Sticky: DIY Skin Care—Recipe Index, Dermarolling, Facial Exercise, thread: http://www.essentialdayspa.com/forum/viewthread.php?p=439158, accessed March 29, 2015.

Feinkel & D. T. Woodley (Eds.), *The biology of the skin.* New York: Parthenon, 2000. Pp. 281–299.

Fernandes, D., 2005. *Minimally invasive percutaneous collagen induction.* Oral Masillofacial Surg Clin N Am 17 (2005) 51-63.

Fife, B. 2004. *The coconut oil miracle.* Penguin Group (USA) Inc.

Fischer-Rizzi, S., 1990. *Complete aromatherapy handbook, essential oils for radiant health*. Sterling Publishing Company New York, NY. 1990.

Fitzpatrick, R. E., 2010. *Fractional resurfacing*. Expert Review of Dermatology 5.3 (June 2010): p269(23). (18720 words) COPYRIGHT 2010 Expert Reviews Ltd.)

Frownies, 2011. *Frownies*. http://www.frownies.com/, accessed July 14, 2011.

Gisquet, 2012. *Most expensive cosmetics*. Forbes.com, accessed January 30, 2012.

Goldberg D.J., Amin S, Russell BA, Phelps R, Kellett N, Reilly LA. , 2006. *Combined 633-nm and 830-nm led treatment of photoaging skin*. Skin Laser and Surgery Specialists of NY/NJ, New York, NY 10022, USA.J Drugs Dermatol. 2006 Sep;5(8):748-53. drdavidgoldberg@skinandlasers.com PMID: 16989189 [PubMed - indexed for MEDLINE] http://www.ncbi.nlm.nih.gov/pubmed/16989189, accessed July 1, 2010.

Goldberg, D. J., Herriot, E. M., 2003. *Secrets of great skin, the definitive guide to anti-aging skin care*. 1st ed. New York, NY: Innova Publishing; 2004.

Gordon, J.R.S, M.D., & Brieva , J.C., M.D., 2012. *Unilateral dermatoheliosis*. N Engl J Med 2012; 366:e25April 19, 2012DOI: 10.1056/NEJMicm1104059

Greek Medicine, 2011. *Greek medicine.* http://www.greekmedicine.net/therapies/Hijama_or_Cupping.html, accessed 7/15/2011. Copyright © 2007 - 2010 by David K. Osborn L. Ac

Guttman, C., 2009. *Percutaneous collagen induction*. Dermatology Times. Cleveland: Aug 2009. Vol. 30, Iss. 8; pg. 58, 3 pgs, Page 1 of 5 http://proquest.umi.com.ezproxy1.library.arizona.edu/pqdweb?ind...=PROD&VType=PQD&RQT=309&VName=PQD&TS=1298747877&clientId=43922, 2/26/11 12:24 PM.

Haneke, Eckart. *Anti-aging medicine world congress*. Expert Review of Dermatology 2.3 (2007): 261+. Health Reference Center Academic. Web. February 26, 2011.

Hampton, A. 1987. *Natural organic hair and skin care*. Organic Press.

http://www.theoilcleansingmethod.com/, accessed September 11, 2010.

Herschthal, J., & Kaufman, J., 2007. *Cutaneous aging: a review of the process and topical therapies*. Expert Review of dermatology 2.6 (Dec 2007): p753(9). (7876 words).

Horrocks, L., 1992. *Natural beauty, total beauty care, using natural ingredients*. Angus and Robertson (an imprint of Harper Collins Publishers).

Kombuchaamerica, 2011. http://www.kombuchaamerica.com/page6.shtml, accessed September 5, 2011.

Kunin, A., 2005. *The DERMAdoctor skinstruction manual*. Simon & Schuster.

Layers of the skin, Copyright Thinkwell, All Rights Reserved. Permission granted on

September 5, 2013.

Lavabre, M., 1990. *Aromatherapy workbook*. Healing Arts Press, Rochester, Vermont.

Lin, FH., et al, 2005. *Ferulic acid stabilizes a solution of vitamins C and E and doubles its photoprotection of skin*. J Invest Dermatol. 2005 Oct;125(4):826-32.

Mahoney, S. 2006. http://www.spafinder.com/Article/245-Getting_Under_Your_ Skin, May / June 2006, accessed March 19, 2011.

Mayo Clinic, 2011. http://www.mayoclinic.com/health/vitamin-e/NS_patient-vita-mine, accessed July 12, 2011.

Merck, 2010. *The merck manuals online medical library*

http://www.merck.com/mmhe/sec18/ch201/ch201b.html, accessed July 5, 2010.

Moore, M., 1989. *Medicinal plants of the desert and canyon west*. Museum of New Mexico Press. 1989.

Monteiro, E.O. & Baumann, L.S., 2006. *The science of cosmeceuticals*. Expert Review of Dermatology 1.3 (June 2006): p379(11). (9025 words).

Mountain Rose, 2011. http://www.mountainroseherbs.com, accessed December 11, 2011.

Natural Health Schools, 2011. http://www.naturalhealthschool.com/acid-alkaline. html, accessed September 5, 2011.

Nature, 2011. *Latest insights into skin hyperpigmentation*. Journal of Investigative Dermatology Symposium Proceedings (2008) **13,** 10–14; doi:10.1038/jidsymp.2008.7 http://www.nature.com/jidsp/journal/v13/n1/full/jidsymp20087a.html, accessed September 18, 2011.

Ndiaye M, Philippe C, Mukhtar H, Ahmad N., 2011. *The grape antioxidant resveratrol for skin disorders: promise, prospects, and challenges*. Arch Biochem Biophys. 2011 Apr 15;508(2):164-70. doi: 10.1016/j.abb.2010.12.030. Epub 2011 Jan 4.

NIH, 2011. Medline Plus, U.S. National Library of Medicine, NIH National Institutes of Health. http://www.nlm.nih.gov/medlineplus/druginfo/natural/940.html, accessed September 17, 2011.

Oprah, 2010. http://www.oprah.com/style/Valerie-Monroes-Guide-To-Serum-Colla-gen-and-Retinoid-Application, accessed June 24, 2013.

Prolight, 2010. http://www.prolightaesthetics.com/catalog/item/6603459/6528796. htmaccessed September 28, 2010.

Puhar, I., Kapudiga, A., Kasaj, A., Willershausen, B., Zafiropoulos, G-G., Bosnjak, A., Plancak, D., 2011. *Efficacy of electrical neuromuscular stimulation in the treatment of chronic periodontitis.* J Periodontal Implant Sci. 2011;41:117-122. doi: 10.5051/jpis.2011.41.3.117.

Sadick, N.S., 2008. *A study to determine the efficacy of a novel handheld light-emitting diode device in the treatment of photoaged skin.* Journal of Cosmetic Dermatology 7.4 (2008): 263+. Health Reference Center Academic. Web. 26 Feb. 2011.

Sauermann, K., Jaspers, S., Koop, U., & Wenck, H., 2004. *Topically applied vitamin C increases the density of dermal papillae in aged human skin.* Research and Development, Beiersdorf AG, Hamburg, Germany author email corresponding author email. BMC Dermatology 2004, 4:13doi:10.1186/1471-5945-4-13. http://www.biomedcentral.com.ezproxy1.library.arizona.edu/1471-5945/4/13.

Self Nutrition Data, 2013. http://nutritiondata.self.com/facts/fats-and-oils/579/2, accessed October 14, 2013.

Sen, C.K., Khanna, S., Roy, S., 2007. *Tocotrienols: vitamin E beyond tocopherols.* Life Sci. 2006 March 27; 78(18): 2088–2098. Published online 2006 February 3. doi: 10.1016/j.lfs.2005.12.001.

Shachtman, N., 2003. *Light at the end of the tunnel.* http://www.wired.com/medtech/health/news/2003/10/60786, accessed October 29, 2003.

Schwanke, J., 2001. *Selenomethionine, vitamin E combo effective.* Dermatology Times. Cleveland: Dec 2001. Vol. 22, Iss. 12; pg. 28, 2 pgs.

Shoulders, M.D., and Raines, R.T., 2009. *Collagen structure and stability.* Annu. Rev. Biochem. 2009. 78:929-958. http://www.biochem.wisc.edu/faculty/raines/lab/pdfs/Shoulders2009a.pdf, accessed July 5, 2013.

Skin Actives, 2011. http://www.skinactives.com/Glucosamine-N-Acetyl.html, accessed September 17, 2011.

Skin Actives, 2011b. http://www.skinactives.com/Hyaluronic-Acid.html, accessed December 11, 2011.

Skin Actives, 2011c. http://www.skinactives.com/Coenzyme-Q10.html, accessed December 11, 2011.

Skin Actives, 2011d. http://www.skinactives.com/Epidermal-Growth-Factor-BT-EGF.html, accessed December 11, 2011.

Skin Actives, 2012. http://www.skinactives.com/Brow-and-Lash-serum-with-KGF.html, accessed January 29, 2012.

Skin Cancer Foundation, 2010. http://www.skincancer.org/understanding-uva-and-uvb.html, accessed September 28, 2010.

Skobe, M., and Detmar, M., 2000. *Structure, function, and molecular control of the skin lymphatic system*. Journal of Investigative Dermatology Symposium Proceedings (2000) **5**, 14–19; doi:10.1046/j.1087-0024.2000.00001.x. Accepted 22 June 2000.

Srinivasan, M., et al, 2006. Ferulic Acid: *Therapeutic potential through its antioxidant property*. J. Clin. Biochem. Nutr., 40, 92-100, March 2007.

Stephanie, 2011. *The oil cleansing method*. http://www.theoilcleansingmethod. com/. The Beauty Bottle, 2011. Accessed May 30, 2011.

Stibich, M., 2010. *Top ten reasons to smile*. http://longevity.about.com/od/lifelong-beauty/tp/smiling.htm, updated February 4,2010. Accessed October 14, 2013.

Tamarkin, D.A., 2011. *How do we get lymph?* http://faculty.stcc.edu/AandP/AP-2pages/Units21to23/immune/lymph.htm. 2011 STCC Foundation Press.

Tourles, S., 1999. *Naturally healthy skin, tips and techniques for a lifetime of radiant skin*. Schoolhouse Road.

Unified Medical Language System (MeSH), 2011. *National library of medicine, genetics home reference*, http://ghr.nlm.nih.gov/glossary=fibroblast, accessed June 26, 2011.

Wagner, K., 2010. *All natural beauty*. http://allnaturalbeauty.us/ani10.htm, accessed July 18, 2010.

Whelan, H.T., M.D., et. al., *The NASA light-emitting diode medical program - progress in space flight and terrestrial applications*. http://www.lumenphoton.com/studies/na-salight.html, accessed March 7, 2011.

APPENDIX A. WEBSITE ADDRESSES

Acids for peels:

Makeup Artist's Choice: www.makeupartistschoice.com

Platinum Skin Care: www.platinumskincare.com

Cupping or Vaculifter:

Store: www.kalinka-store.com/products/291

Ebay: ebay.com, search "cupping"

Amazon: www.amazon.com, search "cupping"

Dry Brushing:

drybrushing.net

www.drweil.com/drw/u/QAA400878/Is-Dry-Brushing-My-Skin-Healthy.html

www.huffingtonpost.com/2012/08/21/dry-skin-brushing-benefits-cellu-lite_n_1811708.html

EMLA numbing cream may be purchased, for example:

Pharmacy Rx World: www.pharmacyrxworld.com/

Facial Exercise:

Resistance

Flex Effect Facial Building: www.flexeffect.com

Ageless if You Dare: www.agelessifyoudare.org

Isometric

Carol Maggio Facercise: www.facercise.com

Cynthia Rowland Beauty Systems: www.cynthiarowland.com

Santa Maria Rungé: www.faceliftingbyexercise.com/author.html

Shape Your Face: www.shapeyourface.com

Beautiful on Raw: www.beautifulonraw.com/raw-food-blog/anti-aging-system/min-dys-journal-being-on-rawsome-flex-program-for-6-weeks/

Scalp

Immortal Hair: immortalhair.forumandco.com/t4383-tom-hagerty-s-scalp-exercises

Hair Loss is Reversible: www.hairloss-reversible.com

Facial Muscle Diagram:

Antranik.org: antranik.org/muscles-of-the-head/

Facial Wrinkle Pads:

Frownies: www.frownies.com

Silc Skin: www.silcskin.com/silcskin/silcskin-facial-pads-brow-set.html

Galvanic/Ultrasound:

Bellaire Industry: www.skinspatula.com/FAQs.htm

Lee Beauty Equipment: www.facialequipment.net/ultrasonic-skin-scrubber-c-9.html

Prolight Aesthetics International:

http://www.prolightaesthetics.com/catalog/item/6603459/6528796.htm

LEDs:

The LightStim Store: store.lightstim.com

Prolight Aesthetics International: www.prolightaesthetics.com/ledlighttreatment.html

Massage:

All Natural Beauty.us: allnaturalbeauty.us/ani10.htm, lymphatic massage

Tutorial: Tanaka Facial Massage: pleasantidleness.wordpress.com/2011/02/06/tutorial-tanaka-facial-massage/

Organic, raw oils:

Mountain Rose Herbs: www.mountainroseherbs.com

Percutaneous Collagen Induction or Dermarolling:

DermaConcepts: www.dermaconcepts.com/documents/0000/0080/Articles_-_medical_needling2.pdf

Microneedle: www.microneedle.com/main/MTS_Roller_PRP_Paper_by_DrGreco.pdf

ENVIRON®: www.environ.co.za/products/medical-roll-cit

Recipes for DIY Skin Care Products:

Essential Day Spa: www.essentialdayspa.com/forum/viewthread.php?tid=11902

Bulk Actives: www.bulkactives.com/formulations.htm

Skin Actives: www.skinactives.com/Skin-Actives-Discussion-Forum.html

Recipe Calculator, calculate amounts of active ingredients to use in recipes

Wholesale suppliesplus : www.wholesalesuppliesplus.com/Calculators/Batch_Size_Calculator.aspx

Bulk Actives: www.bulkactives.com/recipe_creator.htm

Retin-A may be purchased from the internet, for example:

All Day Chemists: www.alldaychemist.com/

Skin Care Message Boards:

Essential Day Spa: www.essentialdayspa.com/forum/

Make Me Heal: messageboards.makemeheal.com/skin-care/

Real Self Skin Care Forum: www.realself.com/skin-care/forum

Skin Care Talk: www.skincaretalk.com

Skin Care Boards: www.skincare.boards.net

Supply Sources for Cosmeceutical and Active Ingredients:

Dr. Clark Store: www.drclarkstore.com

Garden of Wisdom: www.gardenofwisdom.com/home.html

Making Cosmetics: www.makingcosmetics.com

NCN Pro Skin Care: http://ncnskincare.com

Skin Actives: www.skinactives.com

The Herbarie: www.theherbarie.com

The Personal Formulator: www.personalformulator.com/wvss/

Tropical Traditions: www.tropicaltraditions.com

Winter Sun Trading Co.: www.wintersun.com

APPENDIX B. BLENDING SKIN CARE PRODUCTS

DIY skin care products may be prepared by following a recipe or by developing a recipe. Preparing DIY products can be simple or complex depending on the number of active ingredients used and the type of product that is desired.

Follow the formulating guidelines below to prepare high quality DIY skin care products. Key formulating elements include:

- Always prepare DIY skin care products under clean conditions.
- Always wash hands before preparing DIY products.
- Never cross contaminate your active ingredients by accidently blending different active ingredients together. For example, do not use the same measuring utensil for more than one active ingredient.
- Measure all active and inactive ingredients.
- Follow the recommended usage instructions for each active ingredient.
- Wash and dry DIY mixing bowls and utensils between uses.
- Store DIY blended skin care products in new or used, cleaned and sterilized containers.
- Store DIY serums, lotions, or creams in the refrigerator to maintain the strength of the active ingredients and to prevent bacterial growth.
- To prevent an allergic reaction, test your DIY product on a small patch of skin for 24 hours before applying to the face and neck.
- Always wash hands before applying DIY skin care products to the skin.

Tools and items necessary to prepare DIY skin care products:

- A plastic pipette to measure liquids in milliliters.
- A measuring cup that measures small amounts and a larger measuring cup too.
- Several measuring cups and spoons.
- Small glasses, small bowels or cups for mixing.
- Stirring rods or utensils for mixing.
- A funnel to pour the DIY blend into a bottle.
- A scale that measures from 100 grams to 0.01 grams.
- Prepared containers that will be used to store DIY toners and serums; use new, or reuse cleaned and sterilized, brown or green glass bottles with spray or drop tops.
- Prepared containers that will be used to store lotions and creams; newly

purchased two-ounce jars with lids or reused cleaned and sterilized jars and lids.

- Recipes and instructions that include the name of the active ingredient, its concentration, the maximum concentration used for skin care, and the amount required to prepare a one-ounce product.

A new recipe can be developed by calculating the amount of each ingredient based on the desired concentration or by using a blending calculator that may be found on the Internet. DIY skin care recipes are available at online skin care message boards and on the web sites of merchants that sell active ingredients. Write out the recipe or print and file it so that you can use it when you make a new batch. Usage instructions for an active ingredient that is purchased online may be provided with the shipping package or posted on the website of the store where the active was purchased.

When blending a personal formulation, actives are added to a base or carrier such as a toner, serum, lotion, cream, or oil. A store-bought base or a homemade base may be used. For example, to make serums I use aloe vera gel, sea kelp bioferment, or vegetable glycerin diluted with water as my base serum. I then add my active ingredients to this base.

Some active ingredient suppliers provide plastic pipettes or small cups to measure liquids in milliliters. A pipette—similar to a kitchen baster—is used to measure small amounts of liquids. Depending on how the recipe is described, dry ingredients may be measured using measuring spoons or using a small scale that measures weight down to 0.01 grams. You can purchase this type of scale for under $20 dollars.

It is easy to calculate the amount of an active ingredient that will be added to your blend. For example, if using 100 percent pure L-ascorbic acid (LAA) powder:

- Decide the volume of the final product. For example, a one-ounce serum equals 29.6 milliliters (round to 30 for easier calculating)
- Identify the desired concentration of the active ingredient. For example, 15 percent LAA

Commonly used conversion factors for powders and liquids:

> 1 gram = 0.035 ounce
> 1 ounce = 29.6 milliliters (round to 30 ml for calculations)

1 milliliter = 1 gram

When calculating a recipe for a one-ounce serum, 30 ml will be the total or 100% volume. The formulas below use the vitamin C active ingredient to show examples of how to calculate the amount of an active ingredient required to formulate a DIY product. Note that when preparing a LAA serum, other ingredients are necessary to stabilize the blend. A recipe for a LAA vitamin C serum is provided in Appendix D.

To make a 15 percent LAA 30 ml serum:

Use the following conversion formula to calculate the grams of LAA required to prepare a 15 percent concentration vitamin C serum. Assume that the source LAA is pure at 100 percent concentration.

$$\frac{15 \text{ percent LAA}}{100 \text{ percent}} = 0.15 \text{ ounce} * \frac{1 \text{ gram}}{0.035 \text{ ounce}} = 4.3 \text{ grams LAA powder}$$

Add 4.3 grams of LAA powder to 30 ml of a water base.

To make a 20 percent LAA 30 ml serum:

Use the following conversion formula to calculate the grams of LAA required to prepare a 20 percent concentration vitamin C serum. Assume that the source LAA is pure at 100 percent concentration.

$$\frac{20 \text{ percent LAA}}{100 \text{ percent}} = 0.2 \text{ ounce} * \frac{1 \text{ gram}}{0.035 \text{ ounce}} = 5.7 \text{ grams LAA powder}$$

Add 5.7 grams of LAA powder to 30 ml of a water base.

To make a 7 percent tetrahexyldecyl ascorbate (TA) 30 ml serum:

Use the following conversion formula to calculate the milliliters of TA required for a 7 percent concentration 30 ml oil soluble vitamin C serum. Assume that the source is 100 percent TA.

$$\frac{7 \text{ percent TA}}{100 \text{ percent}} = 0.07 \text{ ounce} * \frac{30 \text{ ml}}{1 \text{ ounce}} = 2.1 \text{ ml TA}$$

30 ml serum − 2.1 ml = 27.9 ml oil base

Add 2.1 ml of TA to 27.9 ml of an oil base to make a one-ounce serum.

Use conversion formulas (Appendix C) to determine the amount of each active ingredient to be used in a recipe or use one of the recipe calculators that are available on the Internet.

To make a one-ounce serum with several active ingredients write down each ingredient and the desired concentration of each. Calculate the amount of each active required to achieve the desired concentration for a one-ounce serum. Add up each active ingredient to sum the total volume of the active ingredients and subtract that from 30 ml. Use a base serum for example, water, aloe vera gel, vegetable glycerin, hyaluronic acid solution, or sea kelp bioferment to make up the remaining volume necessary to make a one ounce serum.

The concentration of an active may vary from different suppliers. Follow the usage instructions and blend actives at their recommended concentrations and at concentrations suited to your skin care needs.

There is a wealth of information about active skin care ingredients, DIY skin care recipes, and blending on Internet skin care forums and stores.

APPENDIX C. CONVERSIONS

American Standard to Metric

Capacity:

1/5 teaspoon = 0.98 milliliter (ml)

1 teaspoon = 4.9 ml

1 tablespoon = 14.7 ml

1 fluid ounce = 29.5 ml

Weight

1 fluid ounce = 28.3 grams

Metric to American Standard – metric rounded

Capacity:

~1 ml = 1/5 teaspoon

~5 ml = 1 teaspoon

~15 ml = 1 tablespoon

~30 ml = 1 fluid ounce

100 ml = 3.4 fluid ounces

Weight:

1 gram = .035 ounce

100 grams = 3.5 ounces

APPENDIX D. SAMPLE RECIPES

5 Percent Glucosamine (N-Acetyl Glucosamine or NAG) 2.5 Percent Niacinamide Serum

Glucosamine (n-acetyl glucosamine or NAG)/niacinamide serum increases collagen production and significantly reduces hyperpigmentation, age spots, and uneven melanin distribution when applied to the skin. The recipe provided in Table 2 makes a one-ounce serum.

Blend all ingredients until dissolved and pour into a brown glass bottle. Use every morning before applying lotions, creams, or sunscreen. If you have time, let the glucosamine/niacinamide serum absorb for five minutes before applying vitamin C serum or other products.

Store in the refrigerator.

Ingredient	Concentration (Percent, %)	Amount (Metric)	Amount (American Standard)
Niacinimide	2.5	1.4 grams	1/4 teaspoon
N-Acetyl-Glucosamine (NAG)	5	2 grams	1/2 teaspoon
Water	85	25 milliliter	5 teaspoon
Sea Kelp Biofermament, glycerin, aloe vera gel, hyaluronic acid, vegetable glycerin or water	15	5 milliliter	1 teaspoon

Recipe for glucosamine - niacinimide serum

15 Percent C, E + Ferulic + MSM Serum

Vitamin C, in the L-ascorbic acid (LAA) form, easily degrades when exposed to light and oxygen. Ferulic acid prevents oxidation and stabilizes the LAA. If the vitamin C serum becomes oxidized, it will turn brown and should be disposed of.

The recipe provided in the following table makes a one-ounce serum. Blend water, LAA, MSM, sea kelp bioferment (or hyaluronic acid solution, aloe vera gel, vegetable glycerin, or water) and stir until dissolved. Add the ferulic acid to the vodka and stir until dissolved. Mix the water and alcohol blends. If you like, you may test the blend with pH paper, it should be in the range of 3.0 to 3.5. To raise the pH of the vitamin C serum, add hyaluronic acid solution or sea kelp bioferment. To lower the pH of the serum, add LAA.

Store the final blend in a brown glass dropper bottle and in the refrigerator. Use daily in the morning after applying a glucosamine/niacinamide serum. If you have time, allow the serum to remain on the skin for about five minutes before applying lotions, creams, or sunscreen.

Ingredient	Approximate Concentration (Percent, %)	Amount (Metric)	Amount (American Standard)
L-Ascorbic Acid (LAA) powder	15	4.3 grams	1 teaspoon
MSM powder no fillers	5	1.4 grams	1/2 capsule or 1/2 teaspoon
Ferulic Acid	0.5	0.14 grams	1/2 teaspoon
Vitamin E Oil	1	1.25 milliliter	1/4 teaspoon
Sea Kelp Bioferment Hyaluronic Acid Aloe Vera Gel Vegetable Glycerin or Water	17	5 milliliter	1 teaspoon
Vodka	10	2.5 milliliter	1/2 teaspoon
H2O	7	21.25 milliliter	4-1/4 teaspoon

Recipe for vitamin C serum

APPENDIX E. OIL CLEANSING METHOD

To make the OCM blend, mix castor oil with an oil of your choice, based on your skin type and the qualities that you desire, using the ratios provided in Table 4. Mix a small batch to test the ratio blend that works best for your skin. The higher the concentration of castor oil, the more drying the blend will be.

Oils that can be blended with castor oil for the OCM include, but are not limited to: sesame, olive, jojoba, avocado, or grape seed oil.

Skin Type	Percent Castor Oil	Percent Other Oil
Oily	30	70
Balanced	20	80
Dry	10	90

Oil cleansing method recipe ratios

Made in the USA
Lexington, KY
22 May 2015